Saliva and Salivary Diagnostics

Edited by Sridharan Gokul

Published in London, United Kingdom

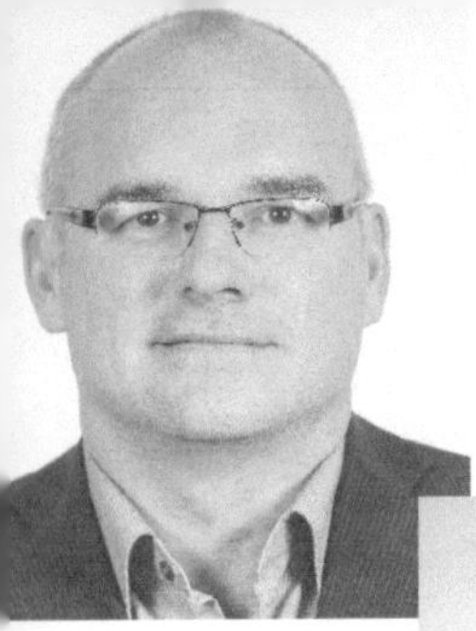
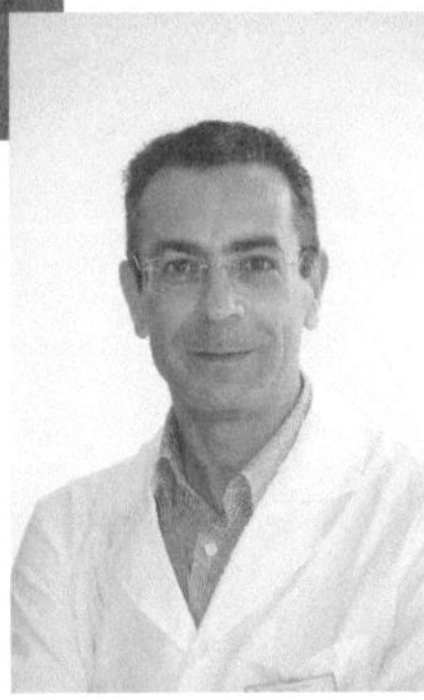
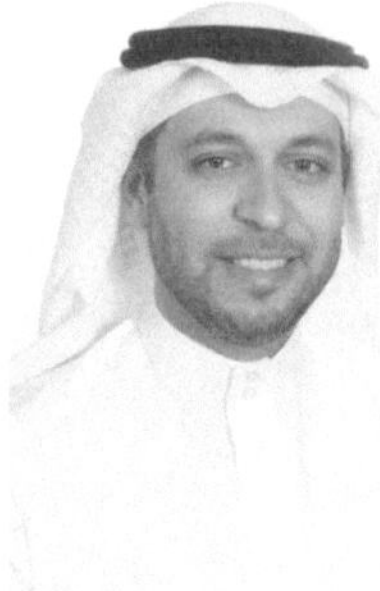
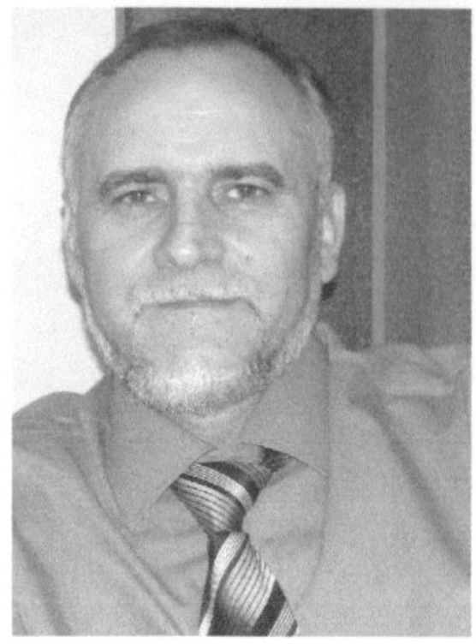
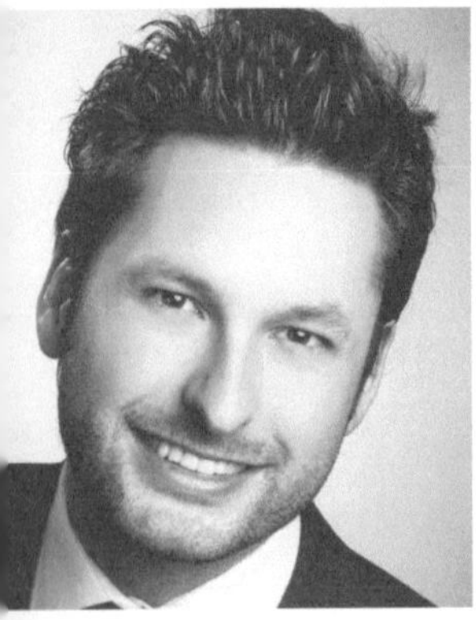
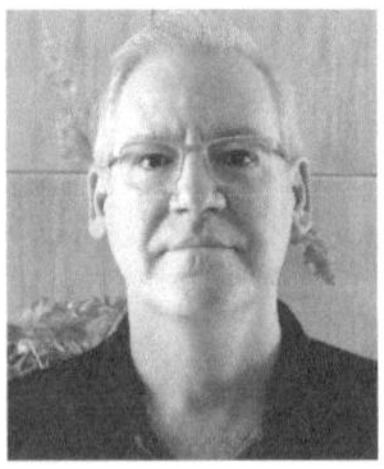
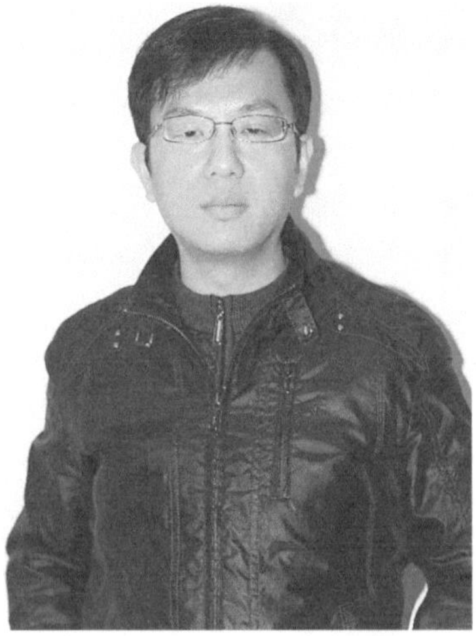

IntechOpen

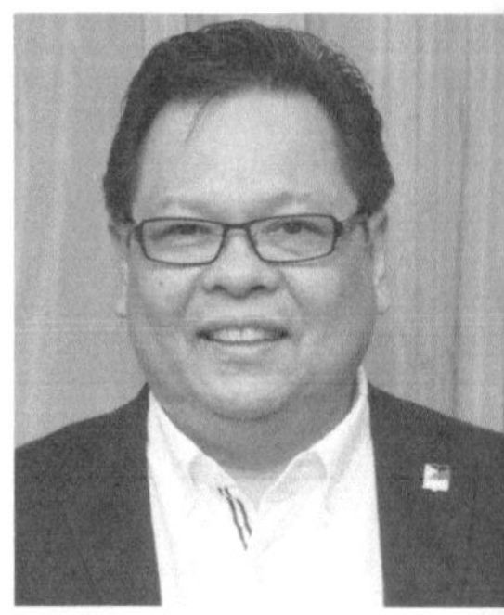
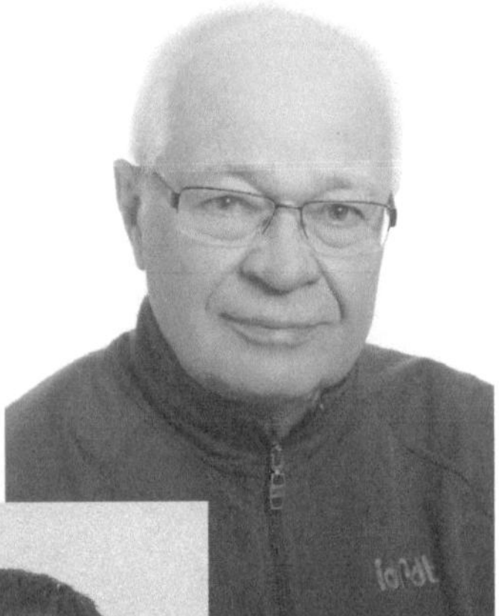
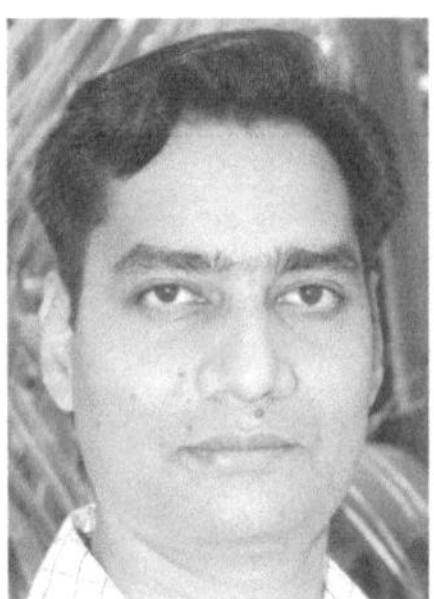
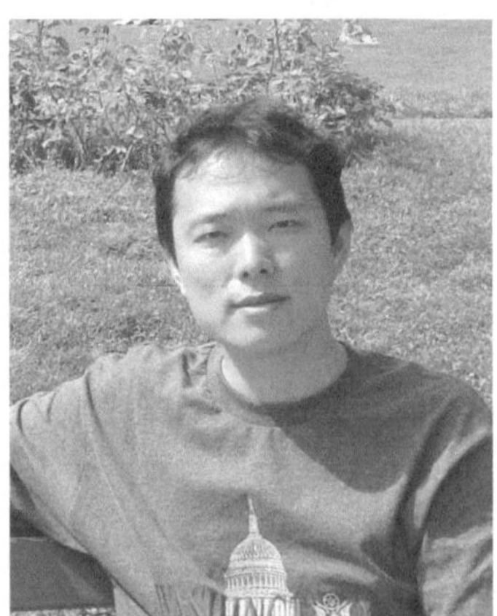
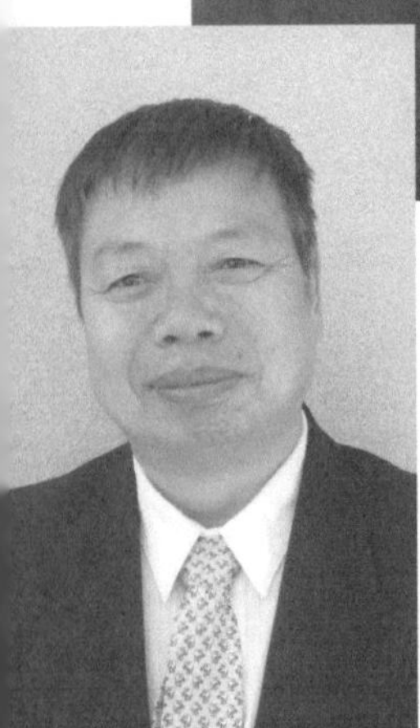
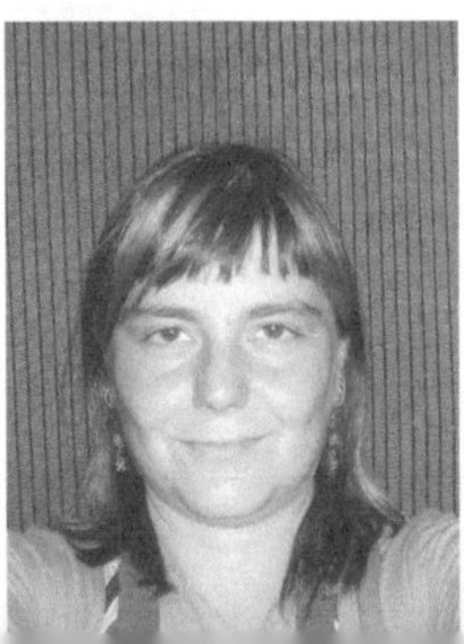

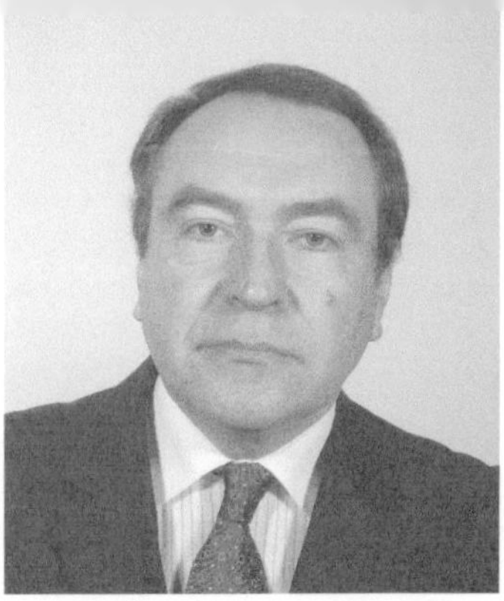
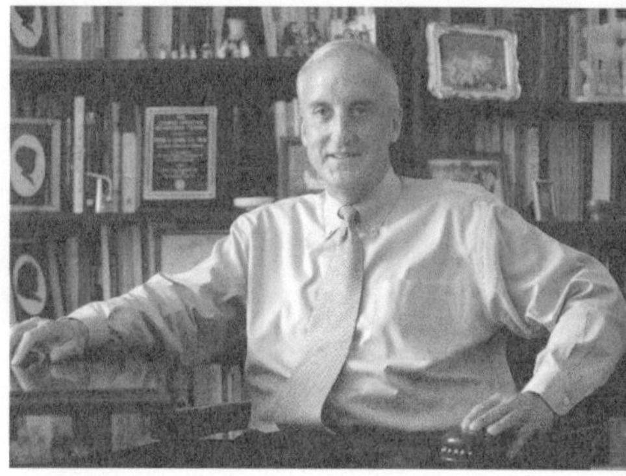
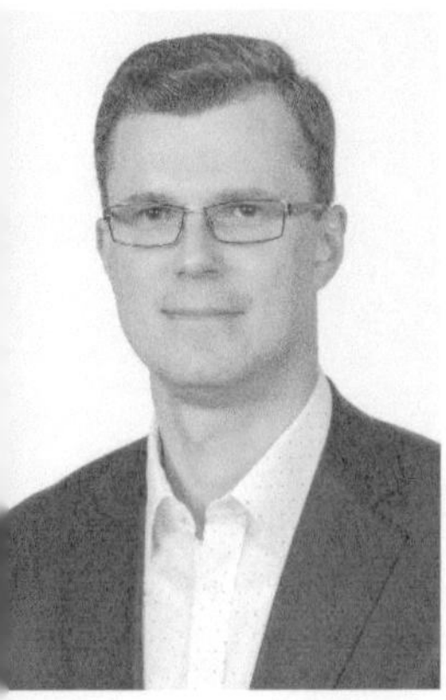
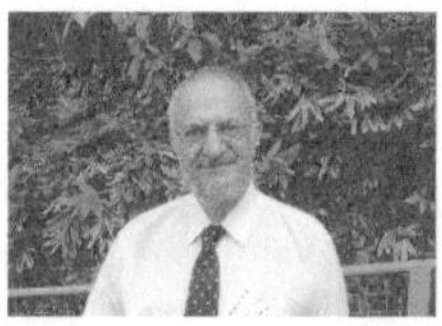
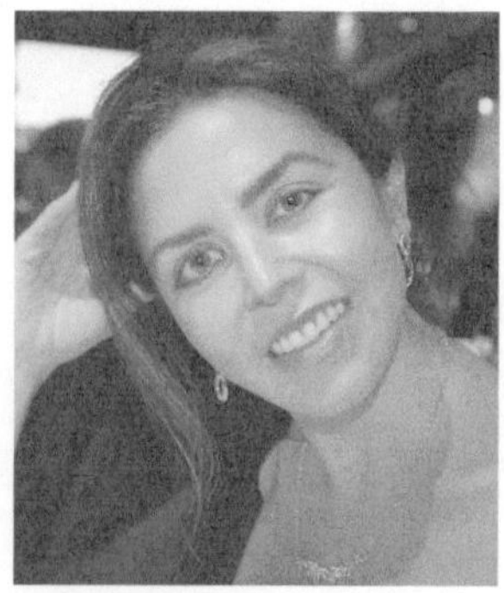

Supporting open minds since 2005

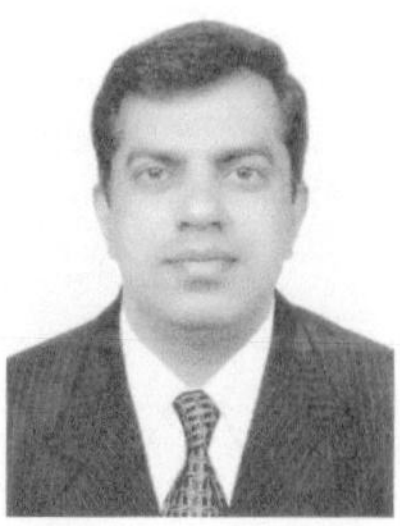
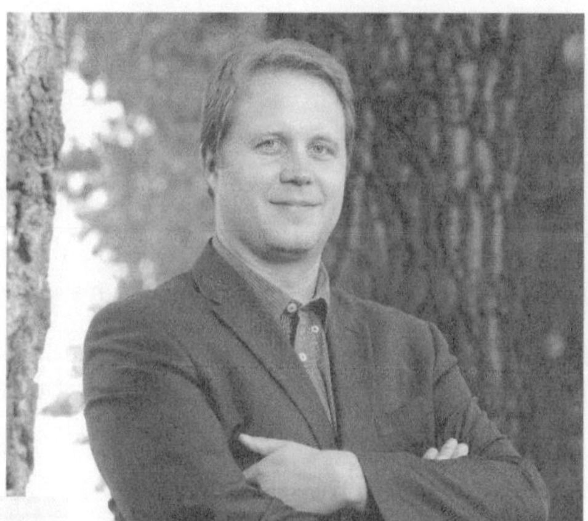
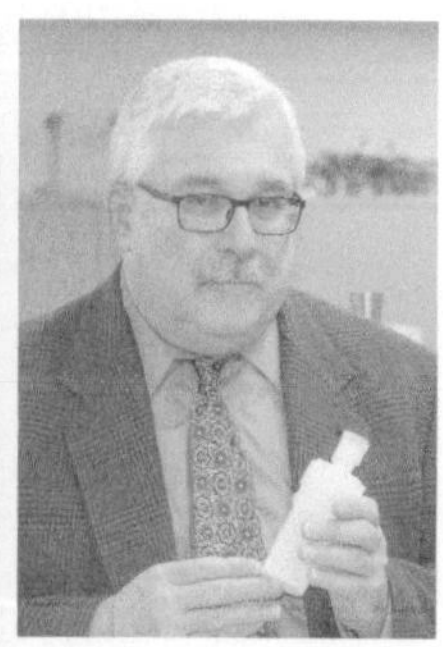
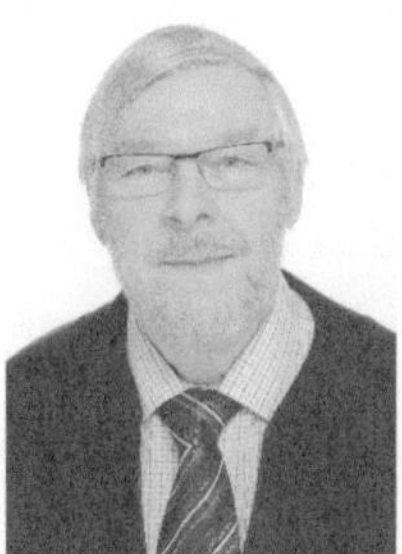
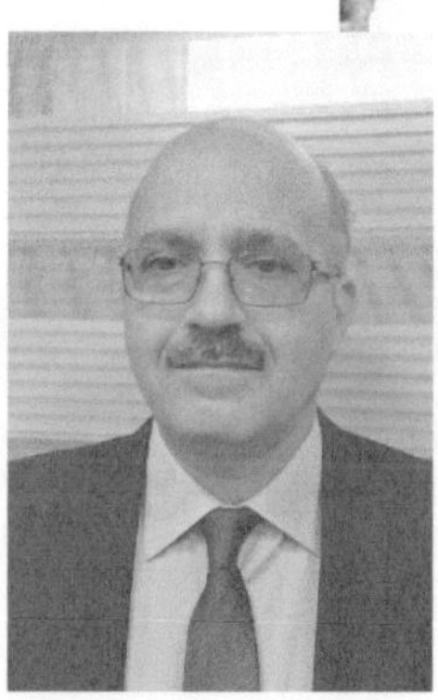
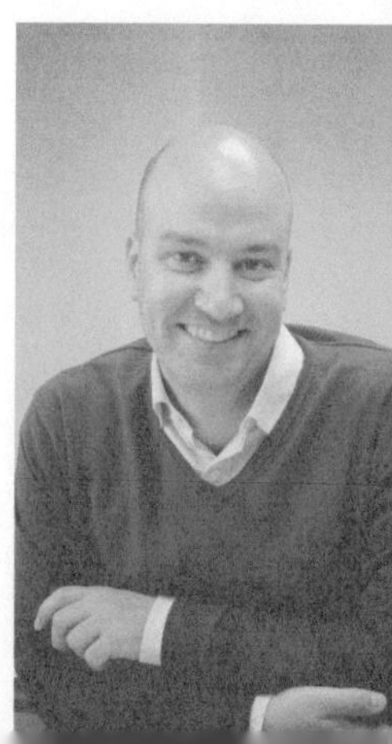
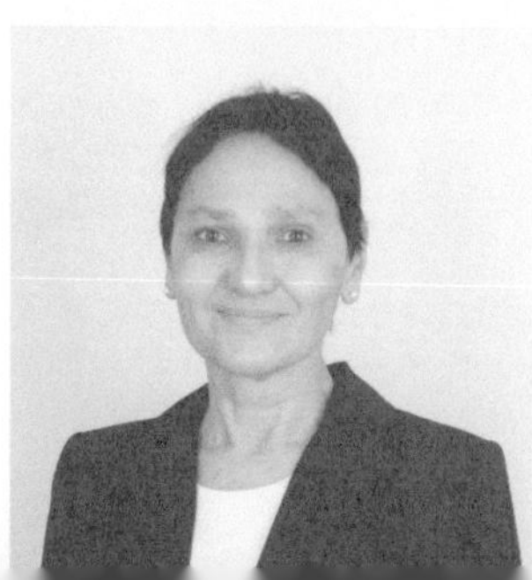

Saliva and Salivary Diagnostics
http://dx.doi.org/10.5772/intechopen.77735
Edited by Sridharan Gokul

Contributors
Charles F. Streckfus, Narendra Maddu, Manohara Bhat, Devikripa Bhat, Varsha Pathiyil, Rahul Udayasankar, Raluca Dumache, Veronica Ciocan, Camelia Muresan, Ramona Parvanescu, Alexandra Enache, Sridharan Gokul

First published in London, United Kingdom, 2019 by IntechOpen
IntechOpen is the global imprint of INTECHOPEN LIMITED, registered in England and Wales, registration number: 11086078, The Shard, 25th floor, 32 London Bridge Street
London, SE19SG – United Kingdom
Printed in Croatia

British Library Cataloguing-in-Publication Data
A catalogue record for this book is available from the British Library

Additional hard and PDF copies can be obtained from orders@intechopen.com

Saliva and Salivary Diagnostics
Edited by Sridharan Gokul
p. cm.
Print ISBN 978-1-78984-309-5
Online ISBN 978-1-78984-310-1
eBook (PDF) ISBN 978-1-83962-390-5

Meet the editor

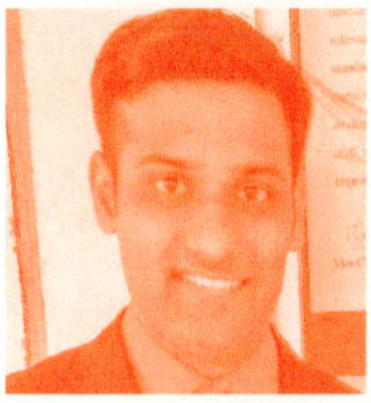

Dr. Gokul Sridharan is an associate professor in the Department of Oral Pathology and Microbiology at YMT Dental College and Hospital, Navi Mumbai. He obtained his PhD for his Thesis "Salivary and Serum Metabolomics in Oral Leukoplakia and Oral Squamous Cell Carcinoma." His fields of interest include oral pre-cancer, oral cancer, salivary diagnostics, oral and maxillofacial diseases, and advanced diagnostic aids with emphasis on bioinformatics and metabolomics. He has several scientific publications and actively contributes as a peer reviewer to numerous journals. He is an active member of the editorial board of several journals of repute. Dr. Sridharan has undergone training and is a qualified diploma holder in medical law and ethics and is also certified in tobacco cessation and control.

Contents

Preface

The health care profession is a dynamic and constantly evolving field periodically encountering new diseases and challenges. The ever-changing facets of human diseases have posed numerous complexities to clinicians and researchers alike. The quest to constantly upgrade the knowledge in dealing with these challenges has resulted in discovery of newer technologies for use in disease diagnosis and treatment.

For decades, the use of blood was widely accepted and depended on for disease diagnosis and treatment formulation. With advancing technologies and understanding of the nature of other body fluids, saliva is rapidly gaining wide importance in diagnosis of not only oral and maxillofacial pathologies but also various systemic diseases. Saliva is a complex fluid containing both organic and inorganic constituents. The multifarious components within saliva not only protect the integrity of oral tissues, but also provide clues to various local and systemic conditions and diseases.

The easy and non-invasive method of saliva collection coupled with the identification of many new salivary components has led researchers from many fields, including dentistry, to believe that saliva could be considered as an attractive diagnostic tool.

Salivary diagnostics has wide applications in the fields of oncology, microbiology, and autoimmunity as well as in various systemic disorders. The anatomical proximity of saliva to various oral lesions makes it an ideal tool for screening and diagnosis of these lesions. Additionally, since saliva is an ultrafiltrate of plasma, it can serve as a diagnostic tool for identifying biomarkers pertaining to various systemic diseases.

The purpose of this project is to understand the physiology of saliva, the methods of saliva collection, and the various analytical methods available as well as emphasize saliva's utility as a dependable body fluid for detection and quantification of disease-specific biomarkers.

Dr. Gokul Sridharan MDS, PhD, PGD (Medical Law and Ethics)
Associate Professor,
Department of Oral Pathology and Microbiology,
YMT Dental College and Hospital,
Kharghar, Navi Mumbai, India

Chapter 1

Introductory Chapter: Saliva - The Future of Disease Diagnostics

Gokul Sridharan

1. Introduction

Saliva is a multi-constituent oral fluid and is considered a mirror of the body's health. The science of saliva has advanced exponentially in the past decade. Saliva and its constituents are being increasingly used for surveillance in various human diseases. The ability to assess the role of salivary components as potential biomarkers is a recent development with increased interest in its use as a diagnostic and prognostic tool [1]. The availability of newer and sensitive technologies has enabled the identification of potential biomarkers even when present in small quantities, thereby signifying the use of saliva as an important assessment media [2].

Salivary diagnostics is an important and significant development in disease diagnosis and treatment delivery. The need for diagnosis of oral and systemic disease and monitoring health regularly is the need of the hour, and saliva owing to its noninvasive and ease of collection along with the ability to detect a myriad of biomarkers is a promising tool. Salivary analytes have been evaluated for their role as potential biomarker in dental caries, periodontal diseases, oral microbial infections such as HIV, autoimmune disorders such as Sjogren's syndrome, drug and hormone monitoring, as well as in diagnosis of systemic diseases. Additionally, salivary diagnostics is emerging as an important investigation in the identification of tumor-specific biomarkers for early detection, diagnosis, prognosis, and therapeutic interventions of oral and oropharyngeal cancers as well as in cancer of distant sites like breast, prostate, cervical, and ovarian cancer. Research is being increasingly undertaken to identify saliva-based biomarkers which either singly or as a panel could be of significant use. Once these biomarkers are quantified and validated, they can be of use in point-of-care diagnostics for chairside detection of various human diseases.

A thorough knowledge of the functions and properties of saliva, its role in health and disease, and the diagnostic technologies available for the identification of saliva biomarkers is of paramount importance to further the knowledge on their usefulness in clinical research and patient management. This formed the basis of the current book on saliva which could serve as an important guide for future research involving salivary diagnostics.

The scientific literature on using saliva as a diagnostic tool begin to emerge since the 1960s. Earlier attempts on the use of salivary diagnostics were confusing owing to the lack of uniformity in the methodology of salivary analysis and the use of available instrumentation. Over a period, the ability to determine salivary components has achieved a sense of uniformity and precision which could be attributed to the understanding of methods of handling saliva samples in various investigating laboratories. The chapters of this book attempt to highlight the advancements of salivary diagnostics over the years, the identification of various salivary-based biomarkers in oral and systemic diseases as evident in the literature, and the future considerations in employing saliva as a diagnostic tool.

 IntechOpen

The book intends to provide an overview of salivary constituents; the functions of saliva; the role of salivary diagnostics in various oral diseases, oral cancer, and breast cancer; and the determination of salivary DNA for forensic analysis.

2. Saliva in health

Saliva is a complex fluid composed of 99.5% water and 0.5% solid material which is inclusive of organic and inorganic constituents. Whole saliva is composed of secretions from the major and minor salivary glands, gingival crevicular fluid, oral mucosal transudate, nasal and pharyngeal secretions, and desquamated epithelial cells. The functions of saliva include but not limited to lubrication, digestion, antimicrobial activity, buffering, and remineralization of tooth enamel. These functions are performed by the different components of saliva [3]. Numerous organic compounds such as proteins, antimicrobials, immunoglobulins, and blood group substances and various inorganic components are present in varying quantities in saliva [4]. The components of saliva are either an inherent component of saliva itself or are derived from blood. The component of plasma may enter into saliva through various processes like ultrafiltration through gap junctions, between cells of secretory units, transudation of plasma compounds into oral cavity through crevicular fluid, and by passive diffusion of lipophilic molecules [2]. The source of information in saliva is largely derived from the variety of DNA, RNA, and proteins present in saliva. Salivary DNA represents the genetic information of the hosting human body, the oral microbiota, and infecting DNA viruses. Salivary RNA provides information on transcription rates of the host genes as well as oral microbiota. Salivary proteins represent genetic information and help understand the translational regulation of the host body [5]. Cell-free saliva has been found to contain over 1000 proteins involved in a wide range of biological functions, mRNA and microRNA transcripts, and metabolites [6].

Specimen collection is an integral part of clinical research for identification and characterization of tumor-related biomarkers. Saliva can be collected under both resting and stimulated conditions. The duration of collecting period is important because flow rates vary with time. It is hence important to follow a standardized collection procedure during the whole sampling period to keep the secretion rate as constant as possible [7]. Further to collection of saliva, it is necessary for appropriate storage of the sample before analysis. The collected saliva should be kept on ice, aliquoted, and frozen as soon as possible to maintain the sample integrity [8]. Certain approaches to store saliva to prevent degradation of salivary compounds include immediate storage without any processing; if analysis is to be done within 30–90 min, saliva can be stored at room temperature; for analysis after 3–6 h after collection, storage is to be done at +4°C; and if analysis is done after days to months after collection, storage is to be done at −20°C or still better at −80°C [2].

The diagnostic techniques employed in the analysis of the processed saliva have made exponential progress over time. Previous techniques for analysis included calorimetric analysis, spectrophotometry, and few optical techniques. These methods have proven efficacy in serum/plasma analysis but did not find similar success in saliva. This could be attributed to the decreased concentration of the various analytes in saliva which demanded a more sensitive and specific technique to enable their identification. The application of liquid chromatography, gas chromatography, flow cytometry, and ELISA was successful in this regard. More recently several techniques such as nuclear magnetic spectroscopy and liquid chromatography coupled with mass spectrometry have been highly successful. Nuclear magnetic resonance spectroscopy enables the identification and simultaneous quantification of a wide range of organic compounds in micromolar range [9]. The advantages of NMR spectroscopy are its high resolution, minimal sample preparation, and time-saving procedure [10]. Mass spectrometry is a method used to analyze samples either directly or following chromatographic or electrophoretic separation [11]. The coupling of liquid chromatography with spectrometry has enabled the identification of low-abundance salivary metabolites with very high sensitivity [12].

3. Saliva as a diagnostic tool

The complex nature of saliva consisting of mixture of components has posed difficulties in identification of specific constituents. However, recent inroads made in the discovery of highly sensitive technologies have enabled the identification of salivary biomarkers with high precision even when present in minute quantities. The role of saliva as a diagnostic tool was evaluated in HIV, oral cancer, as well as in cancer of other sites to name a few.

The need for chairside diagnosis and personalized medicine has led to an increase in the use of fluid-based biomarkers in disease diagnosis and treatment planning. Research involved in identification of disease-specific biomarkers in the blood, urine, and other body fluids was not forthcoming. The lack of absolute success of serum biomarkers along with the improvement in saliva collection and testing presents a unique opportunity for salivary diagnostics.

Molecular alterations are usually attributed to the inherent biological properties of human cell which may contribute to the disease progression. Identification of these alterations can assist in early detection and prediction of prognosis of various diseases including cancer. A comprehensive approach is based on a detection of panel of molecular alteration which can serve as an ideal biomarker for specific diseases. The rapid advancements in the identification of these molecular targets have something to do with the evolution of "omics" group of diagnostic aids [13]. Omics are scientific disciplines constituting the study of related sets of biological molecules. These include genomics, epigenomics, proteomics, transcriptomics, and metabolomics. The term "salivaomics" was coined in 2008 to reflect the rapid development of knowledge about the various omics constituents of saliva [14]. The substantiation of salivaomics technology has led to the discovery, validation, and application of salivary biomarkers in early diagnosis, treatment planning, and prediction of prognosis. Additionally, the development of bioinformatics and statistical tools aids in determining the discriminatory biomarkers in saliva for various oral and systemic diseases [14].

4. Salivaomics

Salivary diagnostics are being extensively reviewed to identify potential biomarkers using these omics technologies [6]. Ever since its discovery, metabolomic investigations can generate quantitative data for metabolites which offers a promising clinical strategy to characterize the association between salivary analytes and a disease [1].

Genomics defines the genetic message and the resulting protein sequences [15]. Genomic analysis in saliva includes the identification of disease-specific characteristics such as somatic mutations in tumor suppressor genes or oncogenes, microsatellite alterations, abnormal protein methylation, and mitochondrial DNA alteration [16]. The proteome represents the complete set of proteins encoded by the genome. Proteomics is the study of proteome that identifies the cellular levels of all the isoforms and posttranslational modifications of the various proteins that are encoded by the genome of the cell under a given set of circumstances [5]. Salivary transcriptomics is defined as the study of the expressed mRNA transcript complement of a cell under different conditions. The large panel of human mRNA is determined using microarray technology followed by validation [17].

Metabolomics is one of the core disciplines of systems biology focusing on the study of low molecular weight organic and inorganic chemicals in biological system [18]. Metabolomics describes the full repertoire of small molecules present in cells, tissues, organs, and biological fluids [6]. The metabolomic profiles can be altered by various pathological processes, and global changes in these profiles may indicate the presence of a disease.

These form the diagnostic alphabets of saliva, and their discovery and quantification have resulted in the application of salivary diagnostics in clinical practice, in point-of-care diagnostics, as well as in personalized medicine.

5. Conclusion

Salivary biomarkers represent an accurate, noninvasive approach for detection of oral and systemic diseases and an attractive area of research. The development of robust and sensitive techniques for detection of salivary biomarkers, its quantification, and validation further maturing to clinical use is the need of the hour. There has been an upsurge in the laboratory-based tests for detection of salivary biomarkers which are ready for definitive validation through the use of various prospective clinical study designs. Researchers can now attempt to develop salivary biomarkers for early detection of diseases employing the omics constituents, saliva-based bioinformatics, and statistical tools. It is worth noting that the technology available enables one to detect promising and new salivary biomarkers as stand-alone tools without relying on their initial identification in the blood and other bodily fluids.

Conflict of interest

The author does not have any conflict of interest to disclose.

Author details

Gokul Sridharan
Department of Oral Pathology and Microbiology, Dr. G. D. Pol Foundation's YMT Dental College and Hospital, Kharghar, Navi Mumbai, India

*Address all correspondence to: drgokuls@gmail.com

References

[1] Spielmann N, Wong DT. Saliva: Diagnostics and therapeutic perspectives. Oral Diseases. 2011;**17**:345-354. DOI: 10.1111/j.1601-0825.2010.01773.xw

[2] Chiappin S, Antonelli G, Gatti R, De Palo EF. Saliva specimen: A new laboratory tool for diagnostic and basic investigation. Clinica Chimica Acta. 207;**383**:30-40. DOI: 10.1016/j.cca.2007.04.011

[3] Cheng YL, Rees T, Wright J. A review of research on salivary biomarkers for oral cancer detection. Clinical and Translational Medicine. 2014;**3**:3-12. DOI: 10.1186/2001-1326-3-3

[4] Kaufman E, Lamster IB. The diagnostic applications of saliva—A review. Critical Reviews in Oral Biology and Medicine. 2002;**13**:197-212

[5] Fabian TK, Fejerdy P, Csermely P. Salivary genomics, transcriptomics and proteomics: The emerging concept of oral ecosystem and their use in the early diagnosis of cancer and other diseases. Current Genomics. 2008;**9**:11-21. DOI: 10.2174/138920208783884900

[6] Bonne NJ, Wong DTW. Salivary biomarker development using genomic, proteomic and metabolomic approaches. Genome Medicine. 2012;**4**:82-93. DOI: 10.1186/gm383

[7] Nurkka A, Obiero J, Kaythy H, Scott AG. Effects of sample collection and storage methods on anti-pneumococcal immunoglobulin A in saliva. Clinical and Diagnostic Laboratory Immunology. 2003;**10**:357-361

[8] Wong DTW. Salivary Proteome Handbook Procedures and Protocols. CA, San Fransisco: National Consortium for Human Saliva Proteome; 2007

[9] Viant MR, Rosenblum ES, Tierdema RS. NMR based metabolomics: A powerful approach for characterizing the effect of environmental stressors on organism health. Environmental Science & Technology. 2003;**37**:4982-4989

[10] Duarte IF, Gil AM. Metabolic signatures of cancer unveiled by NMR spectroscopy of human biofluids. Progress in Nuclear Magnetic Resonance Spectroscopy. 2012;**62**:51-74. DOI: 10.1016/j.pnmrs.2011.11.002

[11] Halket JM, Waterman D, Przyborowska AM, Patel RK, Fraser PD, Bramley PM. Chemical derivatization and mass spectral libraries in metabolic profiling by GC/MS and LC/MS/MS. Journal of Experimental Botany. 2005;**56**:219-243. DOI: 10.1093/jxb/eri069

[12] Zhou B, Xiao JF, Tuli L, Ressom HW. LC-MS-based metabolomics. Molecular BioSystems. 2012;**8**:470-481. DOI: 10.1039/c1mb05350g

[13] Ogino S, King EE, Beck AH, Sherman ME, Milner DA, Giovannucci E. Interdisciplinary education to integrate pathology and epidemiology: Towards molecular and population level health science. American Journal of Epidemiology. 2012;**176**:659-667. DOI: 10.1093/aje/kws226

[14] Wong DTW. Salivaomics. Journal of the American Dental Association (1939). 2012;**143**:19S-24S

[15] Venter JC, Adams MD, Myers EW, Li PW, Mural RJ, Sutton GG. The sequence of the human genome. Science. 2012;**291**:1304-1351. DOI: 10.1126/science.1058040

[16] Zimmerman BG, Park NH, Wong DTW. Genomic targets in saliva. Annals of the New York Academy of Sciences. 2007;**1098**:184-191. DOI: 10.1196/annals.1384.002

[17] Lee Y, Wong DTW. Saliva: An emerging biofluid for early detection of diseases. American Journal of Dentistry. 2009;**22**:241-248

[18] Mamas M, Dunn WB, Neyses L, Goodacre R. The role of metabolites and metabolomics in clinically applicable biomarkers of disease. Archives of Toxicology. 2011;**85**:5-17. DOI: 10.1007/s00204-010-0609-6

Chapter 2

Functions of Saliva

Narendra Maddu

Abstract

Saliva is produced and secreted by salivary glands. The basic secretary units of salivary glands are clusters of acini cells. It is fluid that contains water, electrolytes, mucus, and enzymes, all of which flow out of the acinus into collecting ducts, certainly one of the most important components and an integral component to oral health. The protective role and benefits including buffering, remineralization in the healthy oral mucosa, immune defense, digestion, lubrication, diagnostic purpose, and proteome analysis are fulfilled by saliva. It aids in maintaining mucosal integrity and indigestion through salivary enzymes. The functions of saliva in maintaining oral health and the main factors that cause alterations in salivary secretion and the importance of saliva in caries development and bacterial plaque formation are discussed, and also its role and functions and organic and inorganic constituents in saliva are discussed. This is of great importance in ruminants, which have non-secretory forestomachs. Diseases of the salivary glands and ducts are not uncommon in animals and man, and excessive salivation is a symptom of almost any lesions in the oral cavity.

Keywords: functions of saliva, role of lubrication, antimicrobial functions of saliva

1. Introduction

The secretions of the major and minor salivary glands, together with the gingival crevicular fluid, constitute whole saliva which provides the chemical milieu of the teeth and oral soft tissues [1]. Saliva formation can be evoked by sympathetic and parasympathetic stimulations [2]. The critical function of saliva is required for the preservation and maintenance of oral tissue [3]. Saliva is a complex secretion. About 93% by volume is secreted by the major salivary glands and the remaining 7% by the minor glands. About 99% of saliva is water and the other 1% is composed of organic and inorganic molecules [4]. Saliva consists of both full-length and partially degraded forms of mRNA, and its association with macromolecules may protect salivary RNA from degradation [5]. The proteome of the whole saliva will be relevant to oral health and be crucial for the identification of meaningful biomarkers for oral disease [6]. Sialometry and sialochemistry are used to diagnose systemic illnesses, monitoring general health, and as an indicator of risk for diseases creating a close relation between oral and systemic health [7]. Saliva acts as a mirror of the body's health and could constitute the first line of defense against oxidative stress by controlling and/or modulating oxidative damages in the oral cavity [8].

The analysis of salivary transcriptome may be beneficial effects in the detection of oral cancer and salivary diagnostics [9]. Cationic peptides and other defense proteins like lysozyme, bactericidal–/permeability-increasing protein (BPI), BPI-like proteins, PLUNC (palate lung and nasal epithelial clone) proteins, salivary amylase, cystatins, proline-rich proteins, mucins, peroxidases, and statherin are primarily responsible for innate immunity [10]. The protein and ion components make a solution that is 99% water into a viscoelastic solution capable of many roles, such as acting as a lubricant and an antimicrobial, preventing the dissolution of teeth, aiding digestion, and facilitating taste [11]. With the rapid advancement in salivaomics, saliva, as a noninvasive and safe source, could be a substitute for blood in the diagnosis and prognosis of diseases [12]. Saliva has important functions in maintaining mucosal integrity and indigestion through salivary enzymes, buffering, remineralization, and lubrication [13].

Saliva is an aqueous fluid found in the oral cavity playing a fundamental role in the preservation and maintenance of oral health [14]. Saliva acts in relation to taste, mastication, bolus formation, enzymatic digestion, and swallowing. The protective functions of saliva including maintenance of dental and mucosal integrity indirectly influence the digestive process [15]. The review aimed to discuss the different functions that are performed by the saliva.

1.1 Composition of saliva

Saliva is composed of a variety of electrolytes, including sodium, potassium, calcium, magnesium, bicarbonate, and phosphates. Also found in saliva are immunoglobulins, proteins, enzymes, mucins, and nitrogenous products, such as urea and ammonia. These components interact in related functions in the following general area: (1) bicarbonates, phosphates, and urea act to modulate pH and the buffering capacity of saliva; (2) macromolecule proteins and mucins serve to cleanse, aggregate, and/or attach oral microorganisms and contribute to dental plaque metabolism; (3) calcium, phosphate, and proteins work together as an antisolubility factor and modulate demineralization and remineralization; and (4) immunoglobulins, proteins, and enzymes provide antibacterial action. The components listed above generally occur in small amounts, varying with changes in flow; however they continually provide an array of important functions. It is important to stress that saliva, as a unique biologic fluid, must be considered as a whole that is greater than the sum of its parts [3, 16].

Saliva is a very dilute fluid, composed of more than 99% water. Saliva is not considered an ultrafiltrate of plasma [16, 17]; initially, saliva is isotonic; it is formed in the acini, but it becomes hypotonic when it travels through the duct network. The hypotonicity of unstimulated saliva allows the taste buds to perceive different tastes without being masked by normal plasma sodium levels. Hypotonicity, especially during low-flow periods, also allows for expansion and hydration of mucin glycoproteins, which protectively blanket tissues of the mouth [18]; lower levels of glucose, bicarbonate, and urea in unstimulated saliva augment the hypotonic environment to enhance taste.

1.2 Organic and inorganic constituents of saliva

The organic and inorganic compositions of saliva can supply information about alterations in enzymatic activity in response to periodontal inflammation [19]. Alkaline phosphatase (ALP) is a calcium-phosphate binding protein and a phosphor-hydrolytic enzyme. ALP is considered to be an important indicator of bone formation and is a phenotypic marker for osteoblast cells [20]. ALP was detected in the parotid, submandibular, and minor salivary glands, as well as in desquamated epithelial cells, leucocytes, and bacteria from dental plaque. The presence of the ALP in the saliva and in the gingival crevicular fluid is usually indicative of inflammation and/or destruction of the periodontal tissues. Among the several salivary components, urea is an organic compound that represents the final product of the human catabolism of proteins.

The hydrolysis of urea by bacterial urease enzymes generates ammonia and CO_2 and is considered a major pathway for alkali production in the oral cavity. In addition, ammonia is potentially cytotoxic for the periodontal tissues [21]. Ammonia can increase the permeability of the sulcular epithelium to other antigenic and toxic substances, thereby playing a fundamental role in the initiation of gingivitis [22]. The volume of saliva in the oral cavity depends on several factors, such as stimulation, circadian rhythm, diet, age, drugs, and the hydrogen (H+) ion concentration. Meanwhile, these factors can also be altered due to pathological conditions, such as periodontal disease [23] (**Table 1**).

Salivary component	Function
Amylase	Digestive
Bicarbonate	Buffering
Calcium	Remineralization
Salivary antibodies	Antimicrobial
Lactoferrin	Antimicrobial
Lysozyme	Hydrolysis of cell membrane
Mucins	Digestion, lubrication, and pellicle formation
Protease	Digestion
Water	Mucosal integrity

Table 1.
Components and functions of saliva.

2. Saliva functions

2.1 Immune functions

The components like lysozyme, lactoferrin, salivary peroxidase, myeloperoxidase, and thiocyanate concentrations act as a defense mechanism in the whole saliva [24]. The natural defense properties of salivary secretions through clinical modalities such as the development of (1) diagnostic reagents and tests for local and systemic disease, (2) artificial salivas for the treatment of salivary dysfunction, and (3) topical vaccines to combat against oral diseases [25]. Salivary mucins are well recognized as an important factor in the preservation of the health of the oral cavity and are of significance to the processes occurring within the epithelial perimeter of mucosal defense [26]. Human saliva contains a number of physical, physicochemical, and chemical agents that protect oral tissues against noxious compounds. It effectively removes exogenous and endogenous microorganisms and their products into the gut and continuous presence of both nonimmune and immune factors in the mouth [27]. Salivary mucosal pellicle forms the structural basis of the local innate immune defense mechanism of the oral mucosa [28].

2.2 Saliva proteome analysis

The salivary flow rate influences to a high degree the rate of oral and salivary clearance of bacterial substrates included in foods and snacks [29]. Salivary IgA and lysozyme were inversely correlated with self-perceived work-related stress. As these salivary biomarkers are reflective of the mucosal immunity, results support the inverse relation between stress and mucosal immunity [30]. There was an inverse relationship between the presence of hyaluronidase and the presence of hyaluronidase inhibitors particularly in relation to intraoral wound healing and periodontal disease [31]. Human salivary α-amylase (HSA) is a major secretory protein component of saliva and has important biological functions, including the initial digestion of starch [32]. The collagen-cleaving enzyme matrix metalloproteinase-8 (MMP-8) is present in saliva and acts as measurable indicator of periodontal disease [33].

Amylase present in human saliva was one of the first enzymes to be recognized and molecular mechanisms involved in amylolysis of starch and even of the physiological role of the salivary amylase itself [34]. Lactoferrin in saliva represents an important defense factor against bacterial injuries including those related to *Streptococcus mutans* and periodontopathic bacteria through its ability to decrease bacterial growth, biofilm development, iron overload, reactive oxygen formation, and inflammatory processes [35]. Some defense proteins, like salivary immune globulins and salivary chaperokine HSP70/HSPAs, are involved in both innate and acquired immunities [10]. Lactoferrin is a major component of biologically important mucosal fluids and is essential for mucosal-mediated immunity [36].

The antimicrobial in vitro effects of the salivary proteins lactoferrin and lysozyme on microorganisms is involved in the carious process, obtaining their minimum inhibitory concentration and minimum bactericidal concentration [37]. Salivary alpha-amylase has been proposed as a sensitive noninvasive biomarker for stress-induced changes in the body that reflect the activity of the sympathetic nervous system [38]. Salivary α-amylase levels may therefore serve as an effective indicator in the noninvasive assessment of physical stress [39]. Lactoferrin is a multifunctional mammalian immunity protein that limits microbial growth through sequestration of nutrient iron [40]. Lysozyme in saliva is found to have the antibacterial activity against the pathogen, and there is potential for it to serve an antimicrobial role in the specific application of medical industry [41].

Lactoferrin may be a useful agent to prevent irradiation effects in salivary glands [42]. LTF is examined as a first-line mediator in immune defense and response to pathogenic and nonpathogenic injuries as well as a molecule critical for control of oxidative cell function [43]. Salivary and pancreatic amylases hydrolyze starch and involvement of amylase in adiposity and starch metabolism [44]. Lactoferrin is a secretory protein with various physiological functions, and oral lactoferrin may mitigate psychological stress in humans [45].

2.3 Role of lubrication

The complex mix of salivary constituents provides an effective set of systems for lubricating and protecting the soft and hard tissues [46]. The lubricating and antimicrobial functions of saliva are maintained mainly by resting; saliva results in a flushing effect and the clearance of oral debris and noxious agents [47]. Saliva is a complex fluid, which influences oral health through specific and nonspecific physical and chemical properties [48]. Saliva contains numerous antimicrobial proteins that help protect the oral ecosystem from infectious agent [49]. Proteins can move from blood circulation into salivary glands through active transportation, passive diffusion, or ultrafiltration; some of which are then released into saliva and hence can potentially serve as biomarkers for diseases [50]. Saliva covers the oral hard and soft tissues with a conditioning film which governs the initial attachment of microorganisms, a crucial step in the setup of the oral microflora [51].

2.4 Role of digestion

A high quality of saliva is an essential factor to protect the dental elements against attrition and promote the digestion process [52]. Saliva is the principal fluid component of the external environment of the taste receptor cells which is involved in the transport of taste substances and protection of the taste receptor [53]. The role of human saliva and its compositional elements in relation to the GI functions of taste, mastication, bolus formation, enzymatic digestion, and swallowing [54]. Salivary nonesterified fatty acids (NEFA) are proposed to play a role in oral health and oral fat detection, and they may hold diagnostic and prognostic potential [55].

Lingual lipase generates nonesterified fatty acids (NEFA) from dietary fats during oral processing by lipolysis. Lingual lipase in rodents has strong lipolytic activity and plays a critical role in oral detection of fats [56]. Physiological role of salivary lipolytic activity in the regulation of the basal FFA concentration could be involved in fat taste sensitivity [57]. During chewing, saliva helps in preparing the food bolus by agglomerating the formed particles, and it initiates enzymatic food breakdown [58]. Saliva plays a key role in the eating process and on the perception of flavor. Flavor corresponds to the combined effect of taste sensations, aromatics, and chemical feeling factors evoked by food in the oral cavity [59].

2.5 Role of diagnostic properties

Analysis of saliva may be useful for the diagnosis of hereditary disorders, autoimmune diseases, malignant and infectious diseases, and endocrine disorders, as well as in the assessment of therapeutic levels of drugs and the monitoring of illicit drug use [61]. Fluid addition facilitated chewing of dry foods and feeding disorders caused by hyposalivation [62]. Saliva has been demonstrated to be a promising bodily fluid for early detection of diseases, and salivary diagnostics have exhibited tremendous potential in clinical applications [63]. Saliva has the potential to become a first-line diagnostic sample of choice owing to the advancements in detection technologies coupled with combinations of biomolecules with clinical relevance [64]. Saliva is a useful diagnostic fluid for oral-related diseases. Monitoring salivary biomarkers for oral and systemic diseases could become an important complement to clinical examinations in epidemiological surveys [65] (**Figure 1**).

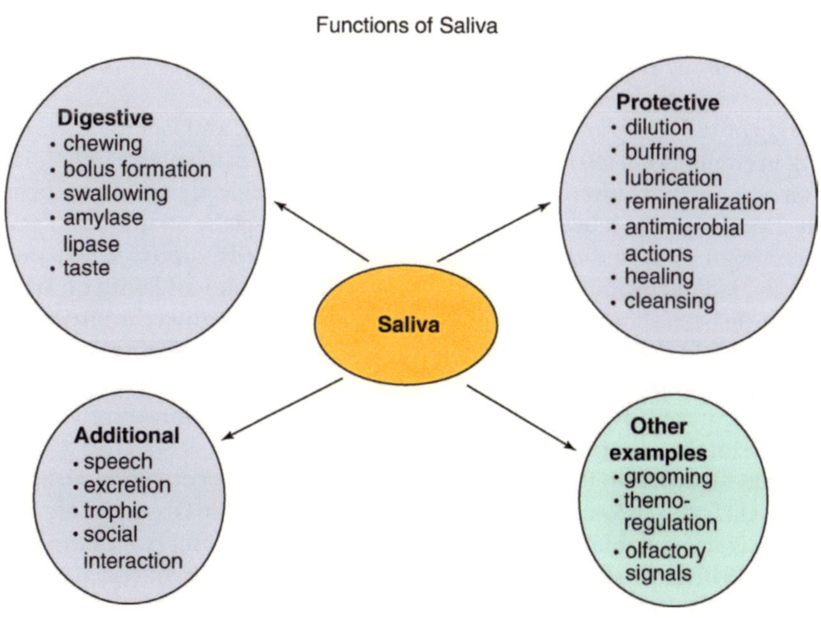

Figure 1.
Different functions of the saliva [60].

The high rate of changes in the composition of saliva can be used for the monitoring of various biorhythms in order to study the physiological characteristics of the human body [66]. The significant influences of the oral environment observed in this study increase the current understanding of the salivary microbiome in caries. These results will be useful for expanding research directions and for improving disease diagnosis, prognosis, and therapy [67].

2.6 Role of maintenance of health teeth

The role of saliva, the prevalence of oral dryness and the consequent importance of salivary flow as well as the relationship between xerostomia and salivary gland hypofunction amongst the causes of oral dryness [68]. Saliva is the medium that bathes the taste receptors in the oral cavity and in which aroma and taste compounds are released when food is eaten. Moreover saliva contains enzymes and molecules that can interact with food [69]. Saliva is an important fluid in the oral cavity as it bathes the teeth and the soft tissues. The salivary pH, buffer capacity and mineral content of calcium (Ca), phosphate (P), sodium (Na), and potassium (K) are important in the tooth de–/remineralization process and calculus formation [70]. Significant change in the pH depends on the severity of the periodontal condition. The salivary pH shows significant changes and thus relevance to the severity of periodontal disease. Salivary pH may thus be used as a quick chairside diagnostic biomarker [71]. Taste perception elicited by food constituents and facilitated by sensory cells in the oral cavity is important for the survival of organisms. In addition to the five basic taste modalities, sweet, umami, bitter, sour, and salty, orosensory perception of stimuli such as fat constituents is intensely investigated [72].

Teeth are exposed to food, drinks, and the microbiota of the mouth and have a high resistance to localized demineralization that is unmatched by bone [73]. The pH of saliva and plaque will result in white spot lesions on the tooth surface which are considered initialization of caries because of demineralization [74]. Saliva is an important biological fluid that aids in mechanically removing food debris and bacteria from the oral cavity and teeth; reduced salivary flow causes ill effects to the oral tissues [13].

2.7 Antimicrobial, antiviral, and antifungal functions

A group of salivary proteins like lysozyme, lactoferrin, and lactoperoxidase working in conjunction with other components of saliva can have an immediate effect on oral bacteria, interfering with their ability to multiply or killing them directly. Lysozyme can cause lysis of bacterial cells, especially *Streptococcus mutans*, by interacting with anions of low charge density chaotropic ions (thiocyanate, perchlorate, iodide, bromide, nitrate, chloride, and fluoride) and with bicarbonate. It has recently been shown that another cationic peptide in saliva the histidine-rich peptide of parotid saliva has growth-inhibitory and bactericidal effects on oral bacteria. The histidine-rich peptides appear to be an effective antifungal agent as well, able to inhibit growth and kill *Candida albicans* at a very low concentration [75].

Lactoferrin, the exocrine gland equivalent of transferrin, is effective against bacteria that require iron for their metabolic processes. It can compete with the bacterial iron-chelating molecules and deprive the bacteria of this essential element. Lactoferrin is also capable of a bactericidal effect that is distinct from simple iron deprivation. Salivary peroxidase is part of an antibacterial system which involves the oxidation of salivary thiocyanate by hydrogen peroxide (generated by oral bacteria) to hypothiocyanite and hypothiocyanous acids. These products, in turn, affect bacterial metabolism (especially acid production) by oxidizing the sulfhydryl groups of the enzymes involved in glycolysis and sugar transport. The antimicrobial effect of salivary peroxidase against *S. mutans* is significantly enhanced by interaction with secretory IgA.

The protective potential of all the antibacterial proteins can be extended by interaction with mucin which can serve to concentrate this defense force at the interface of the mucosa and the inhospitable external environment. When teeth are present, especially if some gingivitis exists, the oral fluids will be augmented by a contribution from the gingival crevice area, the gingival crevicular fluid. This fluid can contribute to the oral defense system by providing (a) serum antibodies against oral bacteria, especially IgG antibodies, (b) phagocytic cells (PMNs), and (c) antibacterial products liberated from the phagocytic cells, e.g., lysozyme, lactoferrin, and myeloperoxidase [27].

The large number of antibacterial and antiviral proteins is present in human saliva. Of interest, most of these antibacterial proteins display antiviral activity, typically against specific viral pathogens. The review focuses on one protein that interacts with both bacteria and viruses, gp340, originally referred to as salivary agglutinin. In the oral cavity, soluble gp340 binds to and aggregates a variety of bacteria, and this is thought to increase bacterial clearance from the mouth. However, when bound to the tooth surface, gp340 promotes bacterial adherence. In the oral cavity, most gp340 proteins are found soluble in saliva and can function as a specific inhibitor of infectivity of HIV-1 and influenza A. In contrast, in the female reproductive track, most gp340 proteins are bound to the cell surface, where it can promote HIV-1 infection [76].

The saliva anti-fungal activity against *Candida albicans* and *Cryptococcus neoformans*. Therefore, the importance of the search for new, broad-spectrum anti-fungals with little or no toxicity cannot be overemphasized. The following properties make histatins promising antifungal therapeutic agents: (1) they have little or no toxicity, (2) they possess high cidal activities against azole-resistant fungal species and most of the fungal species tested, and (3) their candidacidal activity is similar to that of azole-based antifungals. Current research efforts focus on the development of improved histatins with enhanced cidal activity and stability and of suitable and effective histatin delivery systems. These and other approaches may help to outpace the growing list of drug-resistant and opportunistic fungi causing life-threatening, disseminating diseases. The histatins with improved protective properties may also be used as components of artificial saliva for patients with salivary dysfunction [77].

3. Conclusions

Saliva is secreted by salivary glands and has multiple proteins and enzymes. The saliva flow rate and pH are very important for maintenance of oral tissues. The protective role and benefits including buffering, remineralization in the healthy oral mucosa, immune defense, digestion, lubrication, diagnostic purpose, and proteome analysis are fulfilled by saliva. Saliva aids in maintaining mucosal integrity and in digestion through salivary enzymes. Saliva is essential information of the pellicle, which protects the tooth after eruption. Normal salivary composition, flow, and function are extremely important on a daily basis. It occurs in quantities, large or small, and recognition should be given to the many contributions it makes to the preservation and maintenance of health.

Conflict of interest

The authors report no declarations of interest.

Author details

Narendra Maddu
Department of Biochemistry, Sri Krishnadevaraya University, Ananthapuramu, Andhra Pradesh, India

*Address all correspondence to: dr.narendramaddu@gmail.com

References

[1] Edgar WM. Saliva: Its secretion, composition and functions. British Dental Journal. 1992;**172**(8):305-312

[2] Melvin JE. Chloride channels and salivary gland function. Critical Reviews in Oral Biology and Medicine. 1999;**10**(2):199-209

[3] Humphrey SP, Williamson RT. A review of saliva: Normal composition, flow, and function. The Journal of Prosthetic Dentistry. 2001;**85**(2):162-169

[4] Puy CL. The role of saliva in maintaining oral health and as an aid to diagnosis. Medicina Oral, Patología Oral y Cirugía Bucal. 2006;**11**:449-455

[5] Park NJ, Li Y, Yu T, Brinkman BM, Wong DT. Characterization of RNA in saliva. Clinical Chemistry. 2006;**52**(6):988-994

[6] Helmerhorst EJ, Oppenheim FG. Saliva: A dynamic proteome. Journal of Dental Research. 2007;**86**(8):680-693

[7] de Almeida Pdel V, Gregio AM, Machado MA, de Lima AA, Azevedo LR. Saliva composition and functions: A comprehensive review. The Journal of Contemporary Dental Practice. 2008;**9**(3):72-80

[8] Greabu M, Battino M, Mohora M, Totan A, Didilescu A, Spinu T, et al. Saliva-a diagnostic window to the body, both in health and in disease. Journal of Medicine and Life. 2009;**2**(2):124-132

[9] Brinkmann O, Wong DT. Salivary transcriptome biomarkers in oral squamous cell cancer detection. Advances in Clinical Chemistry. 2011;**55**:21-34

[10] Fabian TK, Hermann P, Beck A, Fejerdy P, Fabian G. Salivary defense proteins: Their network and role in innate and acquired oral immunity. International Journal of Molecular Sciences. 2012;**13**(4):4295-4320

[11] Carpenter GH. The secretion, components, and properties of saliva. Annual Review of Food Science and Technology. 2013;**4**:267-276

[12] Zhang CZ, Cheng XQ, Li JY, Zhang P, Yi P, Xu X, et al. Saliva in the diagnosis of diseases. International Journal of Oral Science. 2016;**8**(3):133-137

[13] Kumar B, Kashyap N, Avinash A, Chevvuri R, Sagar MK, Shrikant K. The composition, function and role of saliva in maintaining oral health: A review. International Journal of Contemporary Dental and Medical Reviews. 2017;**2017**:1-6

[14] Milanowski M, Pomastowski P, Ligor T, Buszewski B. Saliva-volatile biomarkers and profiles. Critical Reviews in Analytical Chemistry. 2017;**47**(3):251-266

[15] Pedersen A, Sorensen CE, Proctor GB, Carpenter GH. Salivary functions in mastication, taste and textural perception, swallowing and initial digestion. Oral Diseases. 2018;**24**(8):1399-1416

[16] Dowd FJ. Saliva and dental caries. Dental Clinics of North America. 1999;**43**:579-597

[17] Grant DA, Stern IB, Listgarten MA, editors. Saliva. In: Periodontics. 6th ed. St Louis: CV Mosby; 1988. pp. 135-146

[18] Tabak LA, Levine MJ, Mandel ID, Ellison SA. Role of salivary mucins in the protection of the oral cavity. Journal of Oral Pathology. 1982;**11**:1-17

[19] Todorovic T, Dozic I, Vicente-Barreto M, Ljuskovic B, Pejovic J,

Marjanovic M, et al. Salivary enzymes and periodontal disease. Medicina Oral, Patología Oral y Cirugía Bucal. 2005;**133**:372-378

[20] DEC C, Cohen MM. Mutations affecting bone-forming cells. In: Hall BK, editor. The Osteoblast and Osteocyte. New Jersey: Telford Press; 1990. pp. 431-487

[21] Fure S, Lingström P, Birkhed D. Effect of three months' frequent use of sugar-free chewing gum with and without urea on calculus formation. Journal of Dental Research. 1998;77:1630-1637

[22] Clancy KA, Pearson S, Bowen NH, Burne RA. Characterization of recombinant, ureolytic *Streptococcus* mutans demonstrates an inverse relationship between dental plaque ureolytic capacity and cariogenicity. Infection and Immunity. 2000;**68**:2621-2629

[23] Ghezzi IN, Lange LA. Determination of variation of stimulated salivary flow rates. Journal of Dental Research. 2000;**79**:1874-1878

[24] Saxen L, Tenovuo J, Vilja P. Salivary defense mechanisms in juvenile periodontitis. Acta Odontologica Scandinavica. 1990;**48**:399-407

[25] Levine MJ. Salivary macromolecules. A structure/function synopsis. Annals of the New York Academy of Sciences. 1993;**694**:11-16

[26] Slomiany BL, Murty VL, Piotrowski J, Slomiany A. Salivary mucins in oral mucosal defense. General Pharmacology. 1996;**27**(5):761-771

[27] Tenovuo J. Antimicrobial function of human saliva-how important is it for oral health? Acta Odontologica Scandinavica. 1998;**56**(5):250-256

[28] Kullaa AM, Asikainen P, Herrala M, Ukkonen H, Mikkonen JJ. Microstructure of oral epithelial cells as an underlying basis for salivary mucosal pellicle. Ultrastructural Pathology. 2014;**38**(6):382-386

[29] Lagerlof F, Oliveby A. Caries-protective factors in saliva. Advances in Dental Research. 1994;**8**(2):229-238

[30] Yang Y, Koh D, Ng V, Lee CY, Chan G, Dong F, et al. Self perceived work related stress and the relation with salivary IgA and lysozyme among emergency department nurses. Occupational and Environmental Medicine. 2002;**59**(12):836-841

[31] Pogrel MA, Low MA, Stern R. Hyaluronan (hyaluronic acid) and its regulation in human saliva by hyaluronidase and its inhibitors. Journal of Oral Science. 2003;**45**(2):85-91

[32] Fisher SZ, Govindasamy L, Tu C, Agbandje-McKenna M, Silverman DN, Rajaniemi HJ, et al. Structure of human salivary alpha-amylase crystallized in a C-centered monoclinic space group. Acta Crystallographica. Section F, Structural Biology and Crystallization Communications. 2006;**62**(Pt 2):88-93

[33] Herr AE, Hatch AV, Throckmorton DJ, Tran HM, Brennan JS, Giannobile WV, et al. Microfluidic immunoassays as rapid saliva-based clinical diagnostics. Proceedings of the National Academy of Sciences of the United States of America. 2007;**104**(13):5268-5273

[34] Butterworth PJ, Warren FJ, Ellis PR. Human a-amylase and starch digestion: An interesting marriage. Starch/Starke. 2011;**63**:395-405

[35] Berlutti F, Pilloni A, Pietropaoli M, Polimeni A, Valenti P. Lactoferrin and oral diseases: Current status and perspective in periodontitis. Annali di Stomatologia (Roma). 2011;**2**(3-4):10-18

[36] Alexander DB, Iigo M, Yamauchi K, Suzui M, Tsuda H. Lactoferrin: An alternative view of its role in human

biological fluids. Biochemistry and Cell Biology. 2012;**90**(3):279-306

[37] de Andrade FB, Oliveria JC, Yoshie MT, Guimaraes BM, Goncalves RB, Schwarcz WD. Antimicrobial activity and synergism of lactoferrin and lysozyme against cariogenic microorganisms. Brazilian Dental Journal. 2014;**25**(2):165-169

[38] Sahu GK, Upadhyay S, Panna SM. Salivary alpha amylase activity in human beings of different age groups subjected to psychological stress. Indian Journal of Clinical Biochemistry. 2014;**29**(4):485-490

[39] Koibuchi E, Suzuki Y. Exercise upregulates salivary amylase in humans (Review). Experimental and Therapeutic Medicine. 2014;**7**(4):773-777

[40] Barber MF, Kronenberg Z, Yandell M, Elde NC. Antimicrobial functions of lactoferrin promote genetic conflicts in ancient primates and modern humans. PLoS Genetics. 2016;**12**(5):e1006063

[41] Joel TJ, Suguna SS, Stef SR. Antimicrobial activity of lysozyme against oral pathogens. Asian Journal of Pharmaceutical Research and Health Care. 2016;**8**(2):42-46

[42] Sakai M, Matsushita T, Hoshino R, Ono H, Ikai K, Sakai T. Identification of the protective mechanisms of lactoferrin in the irradiated salivary gland. Scientific Reports. 2017;**7**(1):9753

[43] Kruzel ML, Zimecki M, Actor JK. Lactoferrin in a context of inflammation-induced pathology. Frontiers in Immunology. 2017;**8**:1438

[44] Bonnefond A, Yengo L, Dechaume A, Canouil M, Castelain M, Roger E, et al. Relationship between salivary/pancreatic amylase and body mass index: A systems biology approach. BMC Medicine. 2017;**15**(1):37

[45] Shinjo T, Sakurba K, Nakaniida A, Ishibashi T, Kobayashi M, Aono Y, et al. Oral lactoferrin influences psychological stress in humans: A single-dose administration cross over study. Biomed Reports. 2018;**8**(5):426-432

[46] Mandel ID. The functions of saliva. Journal of Dental Research. 1987;**66**:623-627

[47] Lenander-Lumikari M, Loimaranta V. Saliva and dental caries. Advances in Dental Research. 2000;**14**:40-47

[48] Tiwari M. Science behind human saliva. Journal of Natural Science, Biology and Medicine. 2011;**2**(1):53-58

[49] Glimvall P, Wickstrom C, Jansson H. Elevated levels of salivary lactoferrin, a marker for chronic periodontitis? Journal of Periodontal Research. 2012;**47**(5):655-660

[50] Wang J, Liang Y, Wang Y, Cui J, Liu M, Du W, et al. Computational prediction of human salivary proteins from blood circulation and application to diagnostic biomarker identification. PLoS One. 2013;**8**(11):e80211

[51] van't Hof W, Veerman EC, Nieuw Amerongen AV, Ligtenberg AJ. Antimicrobial defense systems in saliva. Monographs in Oral Science. 2014;**24**:40-51

[52] van Nieuw Amerongen A, Veerman EC. Role of saliva during mastication. Nederlands Tijdschrift voor Tandheelkunde. 1995;**102**(11):441-442

[53] Matsuo R. Role of saliva in the maintenance of taste sensitivity. Critical Reviews in Oral Biology and Medicine. 2000;**11**(2):216-229

[54] Pedersen AM, Bardow A, Beier Jensen S. Saliva and gastrointestinal

functions of taste, mastication, swallowing and digestion. Oral Diseases. 2002;**8**(3):117-129

[55] Kulkarni BV, Wood KV, Mattes RD. Quantitative and qualitative analyses of human salivary NEFA with gas chromatography and mass spectrometry. Frontiers in Physiology. 2012;**3**:328

[56] Kulkarni BV, Mattes RD. Lingual lipase activity in the orosensory detection of fat by humans. American Journal of Physiology. Regulatory, Integrative and Comparative Physiology. 2014;**306**(12):879-885

[57] Neyraud E, Cabaret S, Brignot H, Chabanet C, Laboure H, Guichard E, et al. The basal free fatty acid concentration in human saliva is related to salivary lipolytic activity. Scientific Reports. 2017;**7**(1):5969

[58] Joubert M, Septier C, Brignot H, Salles C, Panouille M, Feron G, et al. Chewing bread: Impact on alpha-amylase secretion and oral digestion. Food & Function. 2017;**8**(2):607-614

[59] Munoz-Gonzalez C, Feron G, Canon F. Main effects of human saliva on flavour perception and the potential contribution to food consumption. The Proceedings of the Nutrition Society. 2018;**77**(4):423-431

[60] Ekstrom J, Khosravani N, Castagnola M, Messana I. Saliva and the control of its secretion. Dysphagia. 2017;**32**:21-57

[61] Kaufman E, Lamster IB. The diagnostic applications of saliva—A review. Critical Reviews in Oral Biology and Medicine. 2002;**13**(2):197-212

[62] Pereira LJ, Gaviao MBD, Engelen L, Van der Bilt A. Mastication and swallowing: Influence of fluid addition to foods. Journal of Applied Oral Science. 2007;**15**(1):55-60

[63] Lee YH, Wong DT. Saliva: An emerging bio fluid for early detection of diseases. American Journal of Dentistry. 2009;**22**(4):241-248

[64] Pfaffe T, Cooper-White J, Beyerlein P, Kostner K, Punyadeera C. Diagnostic potential of saliva: Current state and future applications. Clinical Chemistry. 2011;**57**(5):675-687

[65] Rathnayake N, Akerman S, Klinge B, Lundegren N, Jansson H, Tryselius Y, et al. Salivary biomarkers of oral health: A cross-sectional study. Journal of Clinical Periodontology. 2013;**40**(2):140-147

[66] Belskaya LV, Kosenok VK, Sarf EA. Chronophysiological features of the normal mineral composition of human saliva. Archives of Oral Biology. 2017;**82**:286-292

[67] Zhou J, Jiang N, Wang Z, Li L, Zhang J, Ma R, et al. Influences of pH and iron concentration on the salivary microbiome in individual humans with and without caries. Applied and Environmental Microbiology. 2017;**83**(4):02412-02416

[68] Sreebny LM. Saliva in health and disease: An appraisal and update. International Dental Journal. 2000;**50**(3):140-161

[69] Neyraud E, Palicki O, Schwartz C, Nicklaus S, Feron G. Variability of human saliva composition: Possible relationships with fat perception and liking. Archives of Oral Biology. 2012;**57**(5):556-566

[70] Lavy E, Goldberger D, Friedman M, Steinberg D. pH values and mineral content of saliva in different breeds of dogs. Israel Journal of Veterinary Medicine. 2012;**67**(4)

[71] Baliga S, Muglikar S, Kale R. Salivary pH: A diagnostic biomarker. The Journal of Indian Society of Periodontology. 2013;**17**(4):461-465

[72] Voigt N, Stein J, Galindo MM, Dunkel A, Raguse JD, Meyerhof W, et al. The role of lipolysis in human orosensory fat perception. Journal of Lipid Research. 2014;**55**(5):870-882

[73] Abou Neel EA, Aljabo A, Strange A, Ibrahim S, Coathup M, Young AM, et al. Demineralization-remineralization dynamics in teeth and bone. International Journal of Nanomedicine. 2016;**11**:4743-4763

[74] Bolla VL, Munnangi SR, Manoj Kumar MG, Chowdary UK, Koppulu P, Swapna LA. Correlation between the PH of saliva, plaque and buffering capacity of saliva. International Journal of Applied Dental Sciences. 2017;**3**(4):48-50

[75] Morinushi T, Murayama M, Kinjyo S. Mutans streptococci, Lactobacilli in saliva and acidity for microorganisms in dental plaque: Changes after restorative treatment. The Journal of Indian Society of Periodontology. 2004;**28**:327-332

[76] Malamud D, Abrams WR, Barber CA, Weissman D, Rehtanz M, Golub E. Antiviral activities in human saliva. Advances in Dental Research. 2011;**23**:34-37

[77] Tsai H, Bobek LA. Human salivary histatins: Promising anti-fungal therapeutic agents. Critical Reviews in Oral Biology and Medicine. 1998;**9**:480-497

Chapter 3

Salivary Diagnostics

Varsha Pathiyil and Rahul Udayasankar

Abstract

Saliva is one of the most ideal diagnostic tools. It is inexpensive, noninvasive, and easy to use. Other advantages like ease of collection and minimal patient discomfort make it more acceptable to the patient as well as the clinician. The most challenging aspect in salivary diagnostics is to identify the biomarker that is linked to a disease. Researches are also ongoing to develop a device that can have reliable and valid clinical applications. This chapter briefly discusses the background and current scope of salivary diagnostics, technologies for the discovery of biomarkers along with a summary of salivary sample collection, and processing methods.

Keywords: saliva, metabolomics, proteomics, biomarkers, genomics, epigenomics, sampling

1. Introduction

Saliva is a slightly acidic (pH 6–7) [1, 2] secretory, digestive enzyme that is chiefly produced by the parotid, submandibular, and sublingual glands. These are all paired glands which are serous, mucous, or mixed in their nature of secretions [1–3]. These glands along with other minor salivary glands (labial, buccal, lingual, and palatal) produce approximately 1–1.5 L of saliva per day [1–3].

Functions of saliva [4–6]

- Lubrication of oral tissues and the bolus
- Mechanical cleansing of food and bacteria
- Neutralization of acidic oral constituents
- Antimicrobial activity
- Facilitation of speech, mastication, and swallowing
- Esophageal clearance and gastric buffer
- Digestive functions mediated by enzymes like amylase and lipase
- Healing properties
- Posteruptive maturation of teeth

According to Bricker, diagnosis is the process of evaluating patient's health, as well as the resulting opinions formed by the clinician [7]. Diagnostics can be defined as the art and practice of diagnosis using a series of tests in adjuvant with clinical signs and symptoms. The use of saliva and salivary biomarkers in the diagnosis of various diseases is termed as salivary diagnostics.

Limitations in diagnostics [1, 8]:

- Lack of definitive biomarkers that are specific to diseases
- Lack of an easy and inexpensive sampling method with minimal discomfort
- Lack of easy to use, portable platform to facilitate early disease detection

2. Salivary diagnostics

Saliva has been in use as a diagnostic fluid since the 1960s for conditions like cystic fibrosis [1, 9, 10]. But it was not until the early 1990s that the distinct advantages of saliva over serum were identified [10–12]. For the past two decades, salivary diagnostics have been in use to monitor oral diseases associated with the periodontium as well as dental caries [9, 13]. In the recent past, a vast number of salivary analytes and biomarkers have been discovered that represent various diseases including oral cancer, cardiovascular diseases, various bacterial, and viral infections as well as certain autoimmune disorders. Saliva contains most of the components of serum like hormones, antibodies, growth factors, enzymes, microbes, microbial products, etc. These substances enter saliva through the blood by passive diffusion [1, 8]. Although they are seen only in trace amounts, recent advances in technologies have allowed us to overcome this barrier.

Thus, salivary diagnostics have proven to have a promising future in the diagnostic arena and may offer a quite reliable platform for clinicians to make early clinical diagnosis in the upcoming years.

2.1 Advantages of salivary diagnostics

- Noninvasive, easy to use [8, 9, 14, 15]
- More economical sampling, storage, and shipping compared to serum
- Safer than serum sampling
- Real-time diagnostic value
- Specially trained staff is not necessary
- Any number of samples can be obtained easily
- Collection and screening can be done even outside a clinical setup
- Require less manipulation during diagnostic procedures compared to serum
- Commercial availability of screening assays

2.2 Disadvantages of salivary diagnostics

- Most of the biomarker levels in saliva are lower than that found in the serum. But with advancing technology, this need not be seen as a limitation anymore [8, 15].
- The need for a reliable, sensitive, and specific device that can have valid clinical applications [8].

3. Collection, storage, and processing of salivary samples

Salivary sample can be classified as:

1. Based on the source of saliva
   a. Whole saliva
   b. Specific glandular saliva
2. Based on stimulation for salivation
   a. Stimulated saliva
   b. Unstimulated saliva/passive saliva

It is very important to standardize the methods of salivary collection as several factors influence the quality and the quantity of saliva secreted. The saliva secreted by each gland has characteristics of its own. Variations are observed in the type of protein content as well as in ionic contents. Cystatin C is a biomarker that is found as a submandibular salivary gland-selective protein as it is found in all submandibular fluids but not detected in sublingual gland-specific saliva. MUC5B mucin and calgranulin B, on the other hand, are sub lingual-selective proteins.

The composition of saliva varies according to whether it is basal or stimulated. High flow of saliva has been reported following parasympathetic stimulation with low levels of organic and inorganic compounds.

Low volume of protein-rich and K^+-rich saliva is seen following sympathetic stimulation. Salivary composition is also affected by the presence of food in the mouth. After a meal, total protein and α-amylase in saliva have been seen to increase [16, 17].

3.1 Whole saliva

Whole saliva consists of mainly water and a mix of salivary secretions from all the glands in varying concentrations along with epithelial cells, microbes, and their products [1, 18, 19].

A representation of the entire oral environment, whole saliva is the easiest, feasible, and most convenient mode of salivary sample collection. There is no additional training of the personnel and can even be collected by the study participant.

Whole saliva can be either unstimulated or stimulated. Unstimulated whole saliva is collected by passive drooling or spitting, although care has to be taken to avoid blood and sputum contamination during the spitting method. Studies show that spitting method of salivary sampling contains 14 times more bacteria than when collected by passive drooling. This can influence the storage and further analysis of the sample.

3.2 Stimulated saliva

It is commonly used in patients who have difficulty producing saliva [1, 18, 19]. This method specifically induces salivary production by manual massaging of the gland or with masticatory action such as chewing on paraffin wax, gum, or sterile cotton rolls. Such induction often affects the quantity and pH of the saliva. Use of citric acid specifically lowers the pH of the sample which may interfere with the antibody binding, thus altering the results in hormonal immunoassay. It also interferes with measurement of certain analytes such as testosterone [16].

Chewing on sterile cotton rolls has shown to induce variations in testosterone, DHEA, estradiol, 17-OH hydroxyprogesterone (seen as exceptionally high levels), and S-IgA (maybe seen as exceptionally low). Binding of cortisol to cotton wool fibers is also recorded in literature [16].

There are non-cotton based alternatives such as polystyrene foam swabs, rayon balls, and polyester Salivette. However, studies show that these bind to and remove 87% of progesterone from saliva.

3.2.1 Processing of various salivary samples

Type of sample collected [18]	**Materials required [18]**	**Procedure [18]**
1. Whole saliva	1. 50 ml sterile tube and paper/styrofoam cups 2. Crushed ice and container 3. Distilled water	1. Inform patient of the intended time of saliva collection. Advice to refrain from eating, drinking, or using oral hygiene procedures 1 hour prior to the said time. 2. Time preferred is between 8:00 am and 10:00 am to avoid disturbances due to the circadian rhythm. 3. The subject is asked to rinse well with distilled water for 1 min. 4. 5 min after rinse, the subject is asked to spit into the 50 ml collecting tube. The tube is to be kept in crushed ice between sample collections. 5. Approximately 5 ml of saliva needs to be collected. 6. Processing should occur within 1 hour of collection.
2. Ductal secretion	1. Sterile-modified Carlson-Crittenden/Lashley cup with appropriate PVC tubing 2. Low-affinity conical plastic collecting tubes in ice 3. 5 ml of sterile 20% w/v aqueous citric acid solution (store at room temperature) 4. Cotton tip applicators	1. A modified Carlson-Crittenden tube is positioned near the orifice of the duct 2. Unstimulated saliva is collected for about 15–20 min. 3. Stimulated saliva is collected by intermittent application of 20% aqueous citric acid solution over the dorsum of the tongue.
3. Parotid secretions [18, 20, 21]	1. Sterile-modified Carlson-Crittenden/Lashley cup with appropriate PVC tubing 2. Low-affinity conical plastic collecting tubes in ice 3. 5 ml of sterile 20% w/v aqueous citric acid solution (store at room temperature) 4. Cotton tip applicators	1. A modified Carlson-Crittenden tube is positioned near the orifice of the duct. 2. Unstimulated saliva is collected for about 15–20 min. 3. Stimulated saliva is collected by intermittent application of 20% aqueous citric acid solution over the dorsum of the tongue.

Type of sample collected [18]	Materials required [18]	Procedure [18]
4. Sub mandibular and sublingual secretions [18, 20]	1. Submandibular and sublingual collector (as described by Wolfe et al.) fitted with sterile 100 ml pipette and low-affinity conical plastic collecting tube 2. Distilled water 3. Sterile cotton pads 4. Dental mirror and forceps 5. 5 ml of sterile 20% w/v aqueous citric acid solution (store at room temperature) 6. Cotton tip applicators	Submandibular and sublingual salivary samples are collected separately using the collecting tubes described by Wolfe et al. 1. Subject is asked to rinse with distilled water for 1 min following which cotton pads are place on the floor of the mouth and the buccal mucosa. This is done to prevent contamination from sublingual and parotid secretions. 2. Stimulated saliva is collected using citric acid, by placing the micropipette of the device at the opening of the Wharton's duct. 3. Sublingual saliva is collected in a similar method, except that Wharton's and Stenson's duct orifices are closed with cotton pads.

4. Processing and storage of samples

4.1 Materials required

- Laboratory vortex mixer [18, 21]
- Refrigerated centrifuge able to accommodate 50 ml tubes.
- Cryotubes able to accommodate −80°C temperatures.
- −80°C freezer for long-term storage purposes.
- Aprotinin stored at 4°C (from standard commercial stock solution).
- 400 mM Na_3OV_4 standard stock: 147.12 mg/2 ml water.

Adjust the pH to 10.0. Let the solution boil for about 10 min till it remains colorless. Store at room temperature.

- 10 mg/ml phenylmethylsulfonyl fluoride (PMSF) standard: Dissolve 100 mg PMSF in 10 ml isopropanol by gentle inversion. Store at room temperature.
- SUPERase Inhibitor (Ambion) stored at −20°C.

4.2 Crucial points to remember during sample collection

1. No mucous contamination should be allowed in the salivary sample [18, 19, 21].
2. Sample should be processed as soon as possible after collection and preferably within 1 hour.
3. During stimulated saliva collection, if citric acid is used as stimulant on the dorsal surface of the tongue, lateral surface of the tongue should be swabbed every 30 s.

4. Reduce the number of freeze/thaw cycles to as low as possible to avoid degradation of nucleic acids and proteins.

5. Avoid exposure of sample to air as this may result in oxidation and inactivation of RNAse inhibitors.

4.3 General considerations for salivary storage

1. Saliva fractions are preferred to be stored immediately without any processing [18, 19].
   - Specimens can be stored at room temperature (when analysis is carried out immediately or in 30–90 min from collection).
   - At +4°C (when analysis is carried out in 3–6 h from collection).
   - At −20°C and better at −80°C (when analysis is carried out days to months after collection) [16].

2. Snap freezing of saliva in liquid nitrogen: mix each salivary fraction with 80% glycerol in water in 1:1 ratio, and then dip the sample in liquid nitrogen.
   This inhibits the bacterial protease activity degrading some salivary protein compounds, such as s-IgA.

3. Inhibition of the enzyme activity present in saliva: Mix each salivary fraction with enzyme inhibitors 10:1 (leupeptin, aprotinin, and 4-[2-aminoethyl] benzene sulfonyl fluoride).

A mixture of protease inhibitors and stabilizing substances like aprotinin, leupeptin, antipain, pepstatin A, phenyl methyl sulfonyl fluoride, EDTA, and thimerosal has been documented.

4. Addition of sodium azide (NaN3) to saliva specimens in attempt to retard bacterial growth.

But sodium azide may interfere with horseradish peroxidase, a common component of enzyme immunoassays.

5. Addition of trifluoroacetate at 10% water solution, to denature salivary enzymes that could degrade several salivary compounds, such as proteins and steroid hormones.

6. For protein analysis, the following protease inhibitors are added:

   i. 0.33 μl aprotinin. Invert gently to mix.

   ii. 1 μl Na_3OV_4 (from standard stock of 400 mM). Invert gently to mix.

   iii. 3.3 μl PMSF (standard stock of 10 mg/ml). Invert gently to mix.

For RNA analysis following RNAse inhibitors are added:

- 65 μl of SUPERase Inhibitor (Ambion) stored at −20°C

Samples should be preferably kept on ice, fractioned and frozen as soon as possible to maintain sample integrity. Refrigeration prevents degradation of some of the biomolecules in saliva. Bacterial proteases are seen in saliva which may degrade several salivary proteins and in turn affect protein analyses.

S-IgA can be degraded at room temperature by bacterial protease, while at −30°C a decrease of 10% is seen after 8 months of storage. A 9.2% decrease is seen per month at room temperature which can be avoided by storage at 5°C, for up to 3 months.

4.4 Possible contaminants during saliva sampling

1. Blood: May compromise quantitative estimates of salivary molecules [19, 22].

2. Food products: Steroid antibodies may cross-react with certain food products.

3. Sodium azide: May interfere with procedures like ELISA and EIA.

5. Biomarkers

According to the National Institutes of Health, a biomarker is a characteristic that is objectively measured and evaluated as an indicator of normal biologic processes, pathogenic processes, or pharmaceutical responses to a therapeutic intervention [13, 19].

It is the term given to a change in a biological molecule due to intervention by reactive oxygen, nitrogen, or halide species [23].

5.1 Benchmarks of a biomarker

- A major product of oxidative modification that may be implicated directly in the development of disease [13, 23].

- A stable product, not susceptible to artifactual induction or loss during storage.

- Representative of the balance between oxidative damage generation and clearance (i.e., the steady state but also possibly applicable to the measurement of cumulative oxidative damage).

- Determined by an assay that is specific, sensitive, reproducible, and robust.

- Free of confounding factors from dietary intake.

- Accessible in a target tissue or a valid surrogate tissue such as a leukocyte.

- Measurable within the limits of detection of a reliable analytical procedure.

5.2 Comparison between circulatory and salivary markers

Most of the commonly investigated markers in plasma are seen in a narrow range and is well documented over the years [19]. Due to the novelty of salivary diagnostics, this is a shortcoming, as the markers are still in the process of discovery and documentation. Also, the markers vary through a wide range, quantitatively as well as qualitatively. These variations, physiologically and/or pathologically, make the standardization of salivary analyses a challenge.

Many of the components from plasma reach the saliva mainly through passive diffusion. To compare and reach a successful clinical conclusion, it is important that the concentration of the analyte in the plasma and that in the saliva be highly correlated. Studies have shown that the concentrations of proteins and certain ions are comparable to their level in plasma in a stimulated salivary sample than the sample collected passively.

A number of molecules are produced directly by the salivary glands, which include secretory IgA and lysozyme, the presence of which may be sparse or nil in the respective serum sample. On the other hand, concentration of transferrin, iron, bilirubin, cholesterol, lipoproteins, IgG, and IgM is seen to be 4–15 times more than that seen in saliva.

Certain compounds like blood urea nitrogen, C4, and total bilirubin have high correlation between salivary and serum concentration. This suggests a passive diffusion of these compounds from plasma.

Steroid hormones such as cortisol, cortisone, and testosterone are seen in saliva in their free and unbound state, making salivary analysis a much more preferred method over serum analysis. Although they are also found in their free state in the urine, the sampling of urine is often done and measured over 24 h which is more tedious than salivary sampling.

Nonsteroidal hormones such as melatonin and thyroid hormones can also be analyzed through a salivary sample. However, polypeptide hormones are not as easily detected in saliva due to their large size which hinders in passive diffusion. Plasma leakage through lesions or other modes such as active or facilitated transport may also contribute to detections of polypeptide hormones in saliva.

6. Technologies for discovery of salivary biomarkers

6.1 Proteomic technology

Proteome is the protein component of a genome [1, 8, 24, 25]. Proteomes are found in bodily fluids and are potential sources of disease biomarkers. Proteomics refers to the analysis of the portion of the genome that is expressed. Proteome analysis helps in the identification of any signs of morbidity during early stages of a disease as well as to monitor the progression of the disease. Few analyses used in proteomics are:

- Polyacrylamide gel electrophoresis (PAGE)
- Mass spectrometry (MS)
- Electro spray ionization (ESI)
- Matrix-assisted laser desorption ionization (MALDI)
- Mass analyzers like time-of-flight (TOF), quadrupole TOF, Fourier-transform ion cyclotron resonance (FT-ICR), etc.

Disadvantages: functional changes of the protein may occur due to posttranslational modifications which may affect the reflection of the physiologic or pathologic conditions. To evaluate such posttranslational modifications of proteins as biomarkers, comprehensively analytical methodologies like dendrimer-associated MS/MS, MALDI-MS, and targeted HPLC-ESI-MS/MS are used.

6.2 Transcriptomic technology

Salivary transcriptomes were discovered in 2004 which are basically RNA molecules (mostly mRNA) that are exceptionally stable in saliva [1, 8, 26, 27].

Salivary transcriptome is an emerging concept, and various studies are being conducted all over the world in extraction, purification, amplification, and microarray screening.

Although salivary transcriptomes are still under research, a comparative study done at UCLA regarding accuracy of salivary RNA and serum RNA proved that salivary transcriptomes have a slight upper hand compared to that of serum in certain cases like oral cancer.

As a biomarker, transcriptomes are highly robust and reliable.

6.3 Point-of-care technologies for salivary diagnostics

It includes the application of microfluid and micro/nanoelectromechanical system (MEMS/NEMS) [1, 8, 28]. This is an integrated system that allows the analysis of multiple markers in a drop of the salivary sample, simultaneously with the help of ultrasensitive biosensors. Recently, the UCLA Collaborative Oral Fluid Diagnostic Research Center along with UCLA School of Engineering has developed a MEMS-based electrochemical detection platform that has been named oral fluid nanosensor test (OFNASET) [2, 3]. It is highly specific and sensitive and allows simultaneous detection of multiple salivary analytes and RNA markers [2, 3].

6.4 Metabolomics

Metabolomics has been defined as a global holistic overview of the metabolic status [29]. It facilitates the measurement of comprehensively small metabolites and endogenous markers in bodily fluids and aids in biomarker discovery. Salivary metabolomics has been used successfully in physiology, diagnostics, functional genomics, pharmacology, toxicology, and nutrition.

γ-Aminobutyric acid, phenylalanine, valine, n-eicosanoic acid, and lactic acid have been used in the metabolic profiling of oral squamous cell carcinoma, oral lichen planus, and oral leukoplakia.

GC/MS profiling has proven excellent reproducibility with salivary compounds, such as alcohols, aldehydes, ketones, carboxylic acids, esters, amines, amides, lactones, and hydrocarbons. Reproducibility is an extremely important characteristic in diagnostics that shows way for use of this method to analyze larger sample sizes.

6.5 Salivary microbiome

The microbial population that exists within the oral cavity is collectively referred to as the microbiome [30]. The salivary microbiome provides a unique doorway to analyze the symbiotic and/or pathologic existence between the individual and colonizing microbes. This emerging research field is providing new insights into the functioning of the human immune system and defense mechanisms.

6.6 Salivary genomics

The isolation of high-quality and high-molecular-weight DNA from saliva and its analysis in various clinical purposes can be termed as salivary genomics [30, 31]. Technology has led to the development of various DNA collection kits, stabilizing reagents and purification procedures. These in turn have improved the quantity as well as the quality of DNA comparable to that obtained from blood. The ease of sampling and reliability of the assays have made salivary genomics widely accepted and is opening doors to discovery as well as application of salivary epigenomes in diagnostics.

6.7 Salivary epigenomics

The environmental regulation of the genome and its structural and chemical adaptation without altering the DNA base pair sequence are highlighted by the epigenome [30]. The epigenetic changes such as the length of the telomere, microRNAs, etc. are measurable in saliva. DNA in the blood is derived from a variety of cells including the immune cells, which vary significantly over time. However, contradictory to the DNA obtained in blood, the cellular components as well as the DNA in saliva are representatives of PMNLs and shed epithelial cells of the oral cavity, which are much more homogenous in nature.

Two main epigenetic mechanisms that regulate gene patterns through various tissues are methylation and demethylation of genes. The blood DNA methylation patterns have been noted as highly similar to those that are seen in salivary DNA methylation patterns. The methylation changes have been correlated to a number of systemic diseases including diabetes mellitus, muscular dystrophy, and even early life adversities. It is important in diagnostics, as it shows a map of changes in the human body over a period of time.

7. Salivary biomarkers in various diseases

7.1 Oral squamous cell carcinoma

OSCC has seen an increase in occurrence since the past two decades [13, 17, 32–36]. There has been 5.3 times increase for men and 2 times the increase for women [10]. Several studies have been done to discover and analyze the potential salivary biomarkers for oral cancer [10].

Various salivary biomarkers for OSCC:

- CEA, carcinogenic embryonic carcinogen
- CA19-9, carcino-antigen
- TPS, tissue polypeptide specific antigen
- IGF, growth factor
- MMP-2, MMP-11, metalloproteinase
- HA3, cell proliferation regulator
- CA125, serum tumor marker
- Cyfra 21-1, intermediate filament protein
- IL8, IL 1B DUSP1, chemokine-mediator of inflammatory response
- OAZ1, oncogene
- S100P, polyamine synthesis regulator
- SAT, calcium binding protein, cell cycle, and differentiation regulator polyamine metabolism

- IAP, apoptosis inhibitor
- SCC, squamous cell carcinoma-associated antigen
- RNS, reactive nitrogen species
- 8-OHdG, DNA damage marker
- IgG, immunoglobulin
- Sec IgA, mucosal immunoglobulin
- LOH, loss of heterozygosity loss of specific chromosomal regions
- DNA, hypermethylation gene inactivation

An increase is seen in the following biomarkers in patients with OSCC: carbonyls, lactate dehydrogenase, metalloproteinase-9 (MMP9), Ki67, cyclin D1 (CycD1) [10].

7.1.1 Periodontal diseases

Periodontitis is a group of inflammatory diseases that is characterized by loss of connective tissue [13, 32, 37] attachment and bone around the teeth in conjunction with the formation of periodontal pockets due to the apical migration of the junctional epithelium [32].

Inflammation of the gingiva and periodontal tissues is the first sign of a periodontal disease, usually in response to plaque accumulation [10, 12].

The biomarkers in periodontal diseases can be broadly divided into [32, 37, 38]:

- Inflammatory markers
- Markers of connective tissue destruction
- Markers of bone remodeling

a. Inflammatory markers

- β-glucuronidase—Elevated
- CRP—Elevated
- IL-1β—Elevated
- IL-16—Elevated
- MIP-1α—Elevated in aggressive periodontitis
- TNFα—Elevated

b. Markers of connective tissue destruction

- α2 Macroglobulin—Decreased

- MMP 8—Elevated
- MMP 9—Elevated
- AST—Elevated
- ALT—Elevated
- TIMPs—Decreased

c. Markers for bone remodeling

- Alkaline phosphatase—Elevated
- β C-terminal type 1 collagen telopeptide—Intermediate
- C telopeptide pyridinoline crosslinks of type 1 collagen—Intermediate
- Osteoprotegrin—Elevated
- Osteocalcin—Reduced
- Osteonectin—Reduced
- RANKL—Intermediate
- HGF—Elevated

Some other biomarkers of periodontal disease include [13, 32, 33, 37]:

Fibronectin, elastase, albumin, C-reactive protein, hyaluronic acid, CD44, aspartate aminotransferase, C3 complement

7.2 Biomarkers for breast cancer in saliva

- C-erbB-2 [13, 39]
- VEGF
- EGF
- CEA

7.3 Biomarkers of Sjogren's syndrome

- a-Amylase [13, 40, 41]
- Carbonic anhydrase VI
- Proline-rich proteins (PRPs)
- Prolactin-inducible protein precursor (PIP)

- Lactoferrin b-2- microglobulin
- lg k light chain
- Polymeric Ig receptor

7.4 Biomarkers of cardiac diseases

- Cardiac enzymes like CK-MB, MYO and Tnl [32]
- Inflammatory markers like CRP TNFα MMP-9 and myeloperoxidase
- Adhesion markers like soluble CD40 ligand and slCAM-1

7.5 Biomarkers for HIV

- HIV antibody
- Anti-HIV immunoglobulin [16]

7.6 Biomarkers (transcriptomic) of pancreatic cancer

- KRAS [42, 43]
- MBD3L2
- ACRV1
- CDKL3

7.7 Biomarkers (transcriptomic) of ovarian cancer

- H3F3A [44]
- SRGN
- B2M
- BASP1
- AGPATI
- ILIB
- IER3

7.8 Biomarkers of infectious disease

- Dental caries: presence of *Lactobacillus* sp. and *Streptococcus mutans*
- Candidiasis: presence of *Candida* sp.

- Hepatitis: presence of HBV DNA levels
- Peptic ulcers, gastritis, and cancrum: presence of *H. pylori* [16]

7.9 Pharmaceutical and illicit drugs

- Lithium
- Carbamazepine
- Barbiturates
- Benzodiazepines
- Phenytoin
- Cyclosporine
- Alcohol
- Tobacco
- Marijuana
- Cocaine
- Amphetamines [16]

7.10 Hormones

- Steroidal hormones: cortisol, testosterone, estrogen
- Nonteroidal: melatonin, thyroid hormones [16]

8. Conclusions

Saliva is rightly termed "the mirror of the human body." Saliva is already being used in various scenarios such as investigations for monitoring pharmaceutical as well as illicit drug usage, various malignant neoplasia, hormonal analysis, and even as forensic aids.

The use of saliva as an adjunct to clinical and laboratory investigations in diagnostics is no more a distant dream. The development of more reliable and affordable tests is paving way to a promising future in salivary diagnostics. With increasing awareness towards disease prevention and early diagnosis and intervention, salivary diagnostics could, in the future, be included as a part of routine clinical investigations.

Conflict of interest

None.

Author details

Varsha Pathiyil[1] and Rahul Udayasankar[2]

1 Independent Researcher, Palakkad, India

2 Annoor Dental College Moovattupuzha, Malappuram, India

*Address all correspondence to: varsha1892@gmail.com

References

[1] Lee YH, Wong DT. Saliva: An emerging biofluid for early detection of diseases. American Journal of Dentistry. 2009;**22**(4):241

[2] De Almeida PD, Gregio AM, Machado MA, De Lima AA, Azevedo LR. Saliva composition and functions: A comprehensive review. The Journal of Contemporary Dental Practice. 2008;**9**(3):72-80

[3] Burket LW, Greenberg MS, Glick M. Burket's Oral Medicine: Diagnosis & Treatment. PMPH-USA. Hamilton, USA: BC Decker Inc.; 2003

[4] Pedersen AM, Bardow A, Jensen SB, Nauntofte B. Saliva and gastrointestinal functions of taste, mastication, swallowing and digestion. Oral Diseases. 2002;**8**(3):117-129

[5] Mandel ID. The functions of saliva. Journal of Dental Research. 1987;**66**(1_suppl):623-627

[6] Puy CL. The role of saliva in maintaining oral health and as an aid to diagnosis. Medicina Oral, Patología Oral y Cirugía Bucal. 2006;**11**(5):449-455

[7] Bricker SL, Langlais RP, Miller CS. Oral Diagnosis, Oral Medicine, and Treatment Planning. Philadelphia, USA: Lea & Febiger; 1994

[8] Wong DT. Salivary diagnostics powered by nanotechnologies, proteomics and genomics. The Journal of the American Dental Association. 2006;**137**(3):313-321

[9] Javaid MA, Ahmed AS, Durand R, Tran SD. Saliva as a diagnostic tool for oral and systemic diseases. Journal of Oral Biology and Craniofacial Research. 2016;**6**(1):67-76

[10] Mandel ID, Kutscher A, Denning CR, Thompson RH, Zegarelli EV. Salivary studies in cystic fibrosis. American Journal of Diseases of Children. 1967;**113**(4):431-438

[11] Slavkin HC. Toward molecularly based diagnostics for the oral cavity. The Journal of the American Dental Association. 1998;**129**(8):1138-1143

[12] Mandel ID. A contemporary view of salivary research. Critical Reviews in Oral Biology and Medicine. 1993;**4**(3):599-604

[13] Liu J, Duan Y. Saliva: A potential media for disease diagnostics and monitoring. Oral Oncology. 2012;**48**(7):569-577

[14] Tzioufas AG, Kapsogeorgou EK. Biomarkers: Saliva proteomics is a promising tool to study Sjögren syndrome. Nature Reviews Rheumatology. 2015;**11**(4):202

[15] Krishnamurthy S, Vasudeva SB, Vijayasarathy S. Salivary gland disorders: A comprehensive review. World Journal of Stomatology. 2015;**4**(2):56-71

[16] Lima DP, Diniz DG, Moimaz SA, Sumida DH, Okamoto AC. Saliva: Reflection of the body. International Journal of Infectious Diseases. 2010;**14**(3):e184-e188

[17] D'Cruz AM, Pathiyil V. Histo-pathological differentiation of oral squamous cell carcinoma and salivary lactate dehydrogenase: A biochemical study. South Asian Journal of Cancer. 2015;**4**(2):58

[18] Seymour G, Cullinan M, Heng Nicholas CK. Oral Biology: Molecular Techniques and Applications. Published by Springer, Printed by Humana Press. (E book). 2010

[19] Chiappin S, Antonelli G, Gatti R, Elio F. Saliva specimen: A new

laboratory tool for diagnostic and basic investigation. Clinica Chimica Acta. 2007;**383**(1-2):30-40

[20] Wolf RO. Regulated vacuum system for collecting submaxillary and sublingual saliva. Journal of Dental Research. 1964;**43**(2):303

[21] Heft MW, Baum BJ. Basic biological sciences unstimulated and stimulated parotid salivary flow rate in individuals of different ages. Journal of Dental Research. 1984;**63**(10):1182-1185

[22] Kivlighan KT, Granger DA, Schwartz EB. Blood contamination and the measurement of salivary progesterone and estradiol. Hormones and Behavior. 2005;**47**(3):367-370

[23] Griffiths HR, Møller L, Bartosz G, Bast A, Bertoni-Freddari C, Collins A, et al. Biomarkers. Molecular Aspects of Medicine. 2002;**23**(1-3):101

[24] Helmerhorst EJ, Oppenheim FG. Saliva: A dynamic proteome. Journal of Dental Research. 2007;**86**(8):680-693

[25] Zhang A, Sun H, Wang P, Wang X. Salivary proteomics in biomedical research. Clinica Chimica Acta. 2013;**415**:261-265

[26] Li Y, Zhou X, St. John MA, Wong DT. RNA profiling of cell-free saliva using microarray technology. Journal of Dental Research. 2004;**83**(3):199-203

[27] Park NJ, Li Y, Yu T, Brinkman BM, Wong DT. Characterization of RNA in saliva. Clinical Chemistry. 2006;**52**(6):988-994

[28] Epstein JR, Walt DR. Fluorescence-based fibre optic arrays: A universal platform for sensing. Chemical Society Reviews. 2003;**32**(4):203-214

[29] Zhang A, Sun H, Wang X. Saliva metabolomics opens door to biomarker discovery, disease diagnosis, and treatment. Applied Biochemistry and Biotechnology. 2012;**168**(6):1718-1727

[30] Wren ME, Shirtcliff EA, Drury SS. Not all biofluids are created equal: Chewing over salivary diagnostics and the epigenome. Clinical Therapeutics. 2015;**37**(3):529-539

[31] Fabian TK, Fejerdy P, Csermely P. Salivary genomics, transcriptomics and proteomics: The emerging concept of the oral ecosystem and their use in the early diagnosis of cancer and other diseases. Current Genomics. 2008;**9**(1):11-21

[32] Miller CS, Foley JD, Bailey AL, Campell CL, Humphries RL, Christodoulides N, et al. Current developments in salivary diagnostics. Biomarkers in Medicine. 2010;**4**(1):171-189

[33] Nagler RM. Saliva as a tool for oral cancer diagnosis and prognosis. Oral Oncology. 2009;**45**(12):1006-1010

[34] Cheng YS, Rees T, Wright J. A review of research on salivary biomarkers for oral cancer detection. Clinical and Translational Medicine. 2014;**3**(1):3

[35] Elashoff D, Zhou H, Reiss JK, Wang J, Henson B, Hu S, et al. Pre-validation of salivary biomarkers for oral cancer detection. Cancer Epidemiology and Prevention Biomarkers. 2012

[36] Pathiyil V, D'Cruz AM. Salivary lactate dehydrogenase as a prognostic marker in oral squamous cell carcinoma patients following surgical therapy. Journal of Experimental Therapeutics & Oncology. 2015;**11**(2)

[37] Ozmeric N. Advances in periodontal disease markers. Clinica Chimica Acta. 2004;**343**(1-2):1-6

[38] Miller CS, King CP Jr, Langub MC, Kryscio RJ, Thomas MV. Salivary

biomarkers of existing periodontal disease: A cross-sectional study. The Journal of the American Dental Association. 2006;**137**(3):322-329

[39] Zhang L, Xiao H, Karlan S, Zhou H, Gross J, Elashoff D, et al. Discovery and preclinical validation of salivary transcriptomic and proteomic biomarkers for the non-invasive detection of breast cancer. PLoS One. 2010;**5**(12):e15573

[40] Hu S, Wang J, Meijer J, Ieong S, Xie Y, Yu T, et al. Salivary proteomic and genomic biomarkers for primary Sjögren's syndrome. Arthritis & Rheumatism: Official Journal of the American College of Rheumatology. 2007;**56**(11):3588-3600

[41] Kramer J, Rothstein T. CXCL13 in SJöGren syndrome: A novel biomarker of disease. Oral Surgery, Oral Medicine, Oral Pathology, Oral Radiology, and Endodontics. 2010;**110**(6):e15

[42] Zhang L, Farrell JJ, Zhou H, Elashoff D, Akin D, Park NH, et al. Salivary transcriptomic biomarkers for detection of resectable pancreatic cancer. Gastroenterology. 2010;**138**(3):949-957

[43] Farrell JJ, van Rijnsoever M, Elsaleh H. Early detection markers in pancreas cancer. Cancer Biomarkers. 2005;**1**(2-3):157-175

[44] Lee YH, Kim JH, Zhou H, Kim BW, Wong DT. Salivary transcriptomic biomarkers for detection of ovarian cancer: For serous papillary adenocarcinoma. Journal of Molecular Medicine. 2012;**90**(4):427-434

Chapter 4

Salivary Diagnostics in Oral Diseases

Manohar Bhat and Devikripa Bhat

Abstract

Common oral diseases like dental caries, periodontal diseases and oral cancer have major impact on quality of life. For prevention, treatment and prognosis, it is essential to measure the disease objectively and accurately in a quantitative manner. Quantification of biochemical or molecular specific products of cancers in serum or localized body juices can be one of the current methods of measuring oral diseases objectively. Salivary diagnostics has influenced several researchers and has been verified as an important tool in the diagnosis of many systemic conditions and prognosis of the disease. Developments in the field of molecular biology, salivary genomics and proteomics have directed to the detection of novel molecular markers for oral disease diagnosis, therapeutics and prognosis.

Keywords: oral malignant disorders, dental caries, periodontal disease

1. Introduction

Early diagnosis of the disease, quantification of the disease and prognosis of the treatment are the vital steps in controlling and preventing the diseases that would damage the person's quality of life. Diagnosing these diseased conditions has become challenging and thus necessitates complementing clinical evaluation with laboratory testing [1]. It is essential to have a thorough knowledge in order to control or prevent a disease. When we know the particular clinical, radiological, and histological and laboratory characteristics of the disease, it is easy to prevent the disease condition.

Chronic non-communicable diseases are the major public health problems faced by many of the developed and developing countries in the world. Unlike most of the communicable diseases, chronic non-communicable diseases are initiated by multiple risk-factors. Identifying such risk factors is vital to control the disease burden. Identifying unique compound in the diseased body, which is sensitive and specific to that particular disease can help in identifying and measuring the disease status.

2. Why saliva is used for diagnosis?

Saliva was used as a screening tool for cystic fibrosis in the early 1960s [2, 3]. Saliva is the exudate of serum; hence saliva also contains all the biological compounds like hormones, growth factors, antibodies, enzymes, microbes and their products [2, 4, 5]. Salivary diagnostics has become popular these days as collecting saliva is non-invasive, inexpensive, less technique sensitive and easy to perform as compared to serum.

 IntechOpen

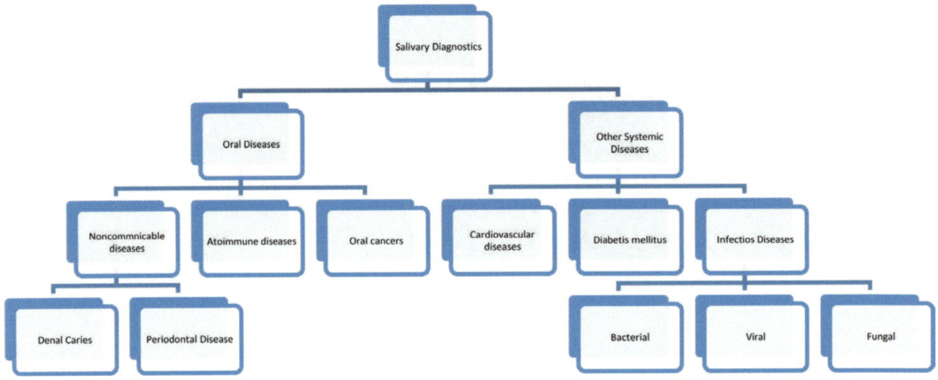

3. Oral diseases

3.1 Dental caries and saliva

Dental caries is a multifactorial oral disease resulting in demineralization of mineralised tissues and denaturation of organic tissues of the teeth initiated by acid production by cariogenic bacteria. These are the major reasons for the loss of teeth among the population. Saliva has protective action in maintaining oral health by its buffering action, antibacterial action and cleansing effect. The awareness of functional properties of saliva as well as those of its distinct components may permit a better valuation of dental caries susceptibility [6].

4. Caries susceptible tests

It refers to intrinsic propensity of the host tissue, the tooth, to be affected by the carious process. It uses saliva as a diagnostic tool in detection and progression of dental caries. Saliva used for caries susceptibility measurement can be explained in four parts:

1. Bacterial count measurement (salivary microbiomics)

2. Colorimetric methods

3. Enzymatic biomarkers

4. Physical property of saliva

5. Bacterial count measurement

5.1 Sampling oral microbial community through saliva (salivary microbiomics)

When considering the hard tissue diseases in oral cavity (dental caries), sampling from the acquired pellicle (AP) provides more sensitive and precise protein profile compared to that of saliva [7–10]. Here saliva plays like carrier of the disease biomarkers.

Only few fractions of known proteins found in human saliva (130/2290 proteins), which are originated from acquired pellicle on dental enamel. The exact biological functions of 51% of known proteins are unknown [8]. This lack of knowledge will provide a new vista to further research.

The particular species of microbial community grow on the AP which is specific to individual oral disease. The quality and quantification of these species can provide a clearer picture on diagnosis and find out the severity of the oral disease.

For example, patients exhibiting dental caries demonstrates dominated acidogenic and acid-tolerant Gram-positive bacteria (i.e., *Streptococcus* and *Lactobacilli* sp) [11].

Some of the salivary determinant tests are as follows

1. *Lactobacillus colony count test*: assessment of the number of acidogenic bacteria can be done by calculating the number of colonies appearing on Tomato peptone agar plates (pH 5.0) after inoculation with a sample of saliva.

2. *Streptococcus mutans level in saliva*: this measures the number of *S. mutans* colony forming units per unit volume of saliva.

3. *Saliva/tongue blade method*: estimation of the number of *S. mutans* in Mutans Salivarius Bacitracin (MSB) agar inoculated by paraffin-stimulated saliva/ Saliva-contaminated wooden spatulas [12].

5.2 Colorimetric methods

1. Snyder's test [7, 13]: the caries susceptibility is correlated with production of acid that is assumed to result due to the fermentation of specific amount of glucose by cariogenic Lactobacillus species by inoculating saliva into agar containing bromocresol green indicator.

2. Albans test: this is a simpler version of Snyder's test in which the patient expectorates directly into tubes that contain the medium. In this test, somewhat softer medium is used that permits the transmission of saliva and acids without the requirement of melting the medium [7].

3. Swab test: the principle of this test is same as that of Snyder's test i.e., capacity of salivary microorganism to form organic acids from a specific carbohydrate medium. The medium encompasses a colour changing indicator dye, bromocresol, which changes its colour when the environment changes its Ph.

5.3 Enzymatic biomarkers

1. *Salivary reductase test*: this test quantifies the activity of the reductase enzyme present in salivary bacteria.

2. *Peroxidase*: peroxidase is a salivary enzyme which neutralises the toxic compound (hydrogen peroxide) produced by oral microorganisms and reduces production of acid in the dental plaque. This severely reduces the plaque accumulation thereby reduces the plaque related diseases like dental caries and periodontal diseases [14].

3. *Collagenase*: it represents in extracellular fluids like serum or saliva represents tissue destruction or cell death. In saliva it indicates destruction of pulp (severe dental caries) or destruction of periodontal tissue [15].

6. Physical properties of saliva

1. Salivary buffer capacity test:

   a. This test measures the amount of millilitres of acid involved in lowering the Ph of saliva via an arbitrary Ph interval, such as, from Ph 7.0 to 6.0 or the quantity of acid or base essential to bring colour indicators to their end point [16].

   b. Population level researches salivary flow rate and buffer effect show a contrary correlation with caries susceptibility [17].

2. Flow rate:

   Many researches showed that, higher the flow rate showed quicker is the salivary clearance [17–19] and greater is the buffer capacity [18] Reduced salivary flow rate and the associated reduction of oral defence systems may cause severe caries and mucosal inflammations [16, 17, 20].

7. Salivary ions

Calcium ion is the most extensively researched salivary ion for dental caries and periodontal disease. Demineralisation of teeth or bone leads to leach out excess of calcium ion into saliva. Increased levels of salivary calcium ion indicate the presence and severity of oral diseases. Similarly increased selenium content in saliva and food is the indicative of dental caries in subjects [21].

8. Periodontal disease and saliva

Diagnosing active phases of periodontal diseases, and identifying those at risk for active disease has been challenging for both clinicians and investigators. Since saliva can be easily collected which contains the locally derived and systemically derived markers of periodontal disease, it can provide specific diagnostic test for periodontitis.

Enzymes present in saliva are contributed by the cells of the salivary glands, oral microorganisms, PMNs, epithelial cells and GCF entering the oral cavity. Studies have shown a reliable relationship between enzyme activity and periodontal status and its response to the periodontal treatment.

Saliva can be categorised in to two types, whole saliva and saliva from specific glands [22–24]. Differences in the amount of fluid and constituents of each gland can be determined in gland specific saliva.

Whole saliva which consists of oral fluids, secretions from the major and minor salivary glands, non-salivary constituents, GCF, bronchial secretions, serum, blood cells, food debris and microorganisms along with their products can also be used as a diagnostic tool.

It has been found that, proposed markers for diseases such as proteins of host origin (i.e., enzymes, Ig), phenotypic markers such as epithelial keratins, host cells, hormones, microorganisms, volatile compounds and ions are found in saliva [25].

Some of the major salivary biomarkers are discussed below:

1. Salivary proteins:

Salivary proteins are formed from combined Direction of DNA and RNAs. Any disparity in DNA or RNA stands can lead to altered protein formation which leads to disease condition and the altered protein becomes the marker of that disease. A patient's salivary protein mapping can provide details on entire body's health because saliva is an exudate of blood and contains juices from gingival crevicular fluid along with major and minor salivary glands, and is much less invasive and more acceptable to the patients compared to blood sampling [10, 26–28] Salivary proteins play a major role in adhesion of microbes on tooth surface through AP formation by stereo-specific mechanism [10, 29]. Salivary proteins can regulate adherence of microorganism by using the carboxylterminal of histatin and of acidic proline-rich proteins (PRPs) by promoting or reducing the attachment to the protein [30–32].

Some of the proteins involved are

A. Enzymes:

  a. Lysozyme

  b. Peroxidase

  c. Collagenase

  d. Acidic and alkaline phosphatase

B. Glycoproteins and proline rich proteins

  a. Dextran

  b. Acquired pellicle forming proteins

  c. Lactic acid and pyruvic acid

  d. Fibronectin

C. Hormones

D. Histatin

E. Matrix metallo proteins

F. Other proteins

  a. Cystatin

  b. Amino acids

  c. Growth factors and vascular endothelial growth factors

A. Salivary enzymes:

  a. *Lysozyme*: lysozyme is an antimicrobial enzyme secreted in human saliva with the ability to hydrolase the 1,4-beta-linkages between *N*-acetylmuramic acid and *N*-acetyl-D-glucosamine existing in peptidoglycan, which is the major component of Gram-positive cell wall. Patients with low levels of lysozyme in saliva are more vulnerable to accumulation of dental plaque, which is considered a risk factor for oral disease and increased salivary lysozyme activity indicates recent infection in oral cavity [33].

b. *Peroxidase*: it inhibits the hydrogen peroxide formation by microbes and there by prevents accumulation of plaque formation. This directly stops the plaque related oral diseases like periodontitis and dental caries. Quantification of this enzyme directly proportional to the severity of the disease status [14].

c. *Collagenase*: collagenase is also known to as MMP-13, is collagenolytic MMP with remarkably extensive substrate specificity. Presence of this in extracellular fluid like serum and saliva indicate tissue destruction or cell death. In saliva this may indicate destruction of periodontal tissue, pulp tissue, infective necrosis or carcinogenic destructions [15].

d. *Acid and alkaline phosphatase*: the enzyme alkaline phosphatase (ALP) and acid phosphatase (ACP) are the twin counterpart enzymes which occur in many organisms ranging from bacteria to man, basically functions by catalysing or blocking the hydrolysis of monoesters of phosphoric acid and also catalyse or block a trans-phosphorylation reaction in the presence of large concentrations of phosphate acceptors [34]. Some researches conveyed amplified activity of acid phosphatase and alkaline phosphatase in the acute stage of periodontal disease, and also observed recovery of enzyme level to the normal range after periodontal therapy [35, 36].

B. Glycoproteins and proline rich proteins:

a. *Dextran*: dextran is a complex, branched glucan (polysaccharide made of many glucose molecules) composed of chains of varying lengths which helps the plaque to attach to the host tissue. Measuring the level of salivary dextran level can helps in calculating the plaque attachment status. There by calculating the plaque related diseases quantitatively [37].

b. *Acquired pellicle forming proteins*: salivary proteins play a chief role in bonding of microbes on tooth surface through acquired pellicle formation by stereospecific mechanism [29]. These salivary proteins decide the type of microbes to grow. Hence identifying these proteins which are specific to grow selective bacteria will provide knowledge about the type of disease.

c. *Fibronectin*: fibronectin is a glycoprotein that mediates adhesion between cells and encourages selective adhesion and colonisation of certain favourable bacterial species. It also involved in inflammation, chemotaxis, and wound healing and tissue repair [23, 38]. Quantification of fibronectin in saliva provides a clear picture on periodontal disease status.

C. Hormones:

Cortisol: cortisol is a hormone highly sensitive to emotional changes and is stress related. It provides anti-inflammatory and immunosuppressive effect. This has direct effect on oral infection and dental plaque related illness [38, 39]. Even though lots of researches indicate the relation of cortisol and oral diseases, more specific and confirmatory researches are needed.

D. Histatin:

Histatin is a salivary protein secreted from parotid and submandibular glands with definite antimicrobial properties. It interacts with endotoxic lipopolysaccharides situated in the membrane of Gram-negative bacteria and neutralises it. It also has antihistaminic action, hence influences oral inflammation [38, 40, 41].

E. Matrix metallo proteins:

They are host proteinases accountable for both tissue degradation and remodelling. The presence of these metallo proteins indicates tissue destruction. MMP 8 is the most predominant MMP found in ill periodontal tissue and GCF. Recent researches reviled that the level of MMP-8 was highly raised in saliva of patients with periodontal disease [38, 42].

F. Other proteins:

a. *Cystatin:* this is a proteolytic enzyme produced by pathogenic bacteria, inflammatory cells, fibroblasts and osteoclasts which have collagenolytic property. It helps in spreading of oral disease to different planes also progress the disease status [23, 38]. Measuring the level in saliva can explain the severity of the oral diseases like periodontal disease and potentially malignant disease.

b. *Amino acids:* some of the amino acids like Proline shows increased levels in saliva of periodontally ill subjects compared to the healthy individuals. This may be due to degradation of salivary proteins by bacterial activities [38, 43, 44]. Presence of proline in saliva directly proportional to the level of bacteria in dental plaque. Hence it quantifies the plaque related oral diseases.

c. *Growth factors and vascular endothelial growth factors:* these are angiogenic cytokines associated with inflammation and healing tissue. Higher level of these proteins in saliva observed in the inflammatory conditions (periodontal diseases) or growth of tumour (Malignant tumours) [23, 38].

G. Human salivary immune system:

a. *Immunoglobulins*: immunoglobulins are specific first-line defence mechanism of saliva. The chief immunoglobulin in saliva is secretory IgA (sIgA), which is produced by the plasma cells in the salivary glands. IgA has 2 subclasses, IgA1 which is predominated in serum and IgA2, which is predominantly present in secretions like saliva, milk and sweats [38, 45]. Many researches show the positive correlation between severity of inflammation (Periodontal disease) and IgA concentration [14, 46].

b. *Salivary neutrophil count*: neutrophils play a major role in the innate immune response. Most of the oral diseases are associated with infection and inflammations, which are explained in the form of neutrophil count in saliva. Very meagre research directed to correlate the neutrophils in plaque, saliva, and gingival crevicular fluid (GCF) to periodontally healthy and diseased subjects. These researches reviled that there is positive correlation between oral diseases with PMN counts [47–49].

H. Salivary ions:

Calcium ion in saliva indicates demineralization of teeth or alveolar bone which leaches out into saliva indicating severity of dental and periodontal diseases [21].

I. Oxidative stress assessment:

Redox (reduction and oxidation) reactions are common in all cells. But imbalance between reduction and oxidation process can lead to oxidative stress within the cell which destroys the cell. Oxidative stress was involved in the progression of periodontal diseases [50–52]. In chronic periodontitis, there was lower serum total antioxidant level when equated to the control individuals [52, 53] Biomarkers of lipid peroxidation (one of the oxidative stress-mediated pathways) such as 8-isoprostane and malondialdehyde (MDA) were elevated in patients with chronic periodontitis [52, 54–56].

J. Salivary Microbiomics:

The particular species of microbial community grow on the AP which is specific to individual oral disease. The quality and quantification of these species can provide a clearer picture on diagnosis and find out the severity of the oral disease. Patients with periodontal disease Express increased percentage of obligately anaerobic bacteria (i.e., Gram-negative species) [10, 57].

Some of the literatures on salivary biomarkers to detect periodontal diseases are as follows:

Author (year)	Biomarkers	Inference
Nakamura and Slots (1983) [35]	Salivary enzymes	Significant difference between diseases and healthy periodontium. No significant difference between LJP and AP
Zambon et al. (1985) [58]	levels of caprylate esterase lipase, leucine, valine and cysteine aminopeptidases, trypsin, B-galactosidase, B-glucuronidase and B-glucosidase, sub gingival black pigmented bacteroides and motile organisms	A decrease was seen in the levels of all the biomarkers after the treatment in AP
Gregory et al. (1992) [59]	Immunoglobulins	Igs in LPJ patients was higher than healthy individuals of same age, race and gender
Gibbons et al. (1986) [30]	Fibronectin-degrading enzymes in saliva	This biomarker was higher in concentration in diseased patients
Nieminem et al. (1993) [60]	Protease levels	Decrease in the levels of protease markers after the treatment in advanced periodontitis
Ingman et al. 1993 [61]	Collagenase, elastase like and trypsin like activity	AP patients' saliva demonstrated a higher level of protease, collagenase and elastase lie activity when compared to LJP and healthy patients
Uitto et al. (1990) [62]	Collagenase	Higher in periodontitis patients
Orner 1976 [63] Halinen et al. 1996 [64]	Collagenase, activated matrix metalloproteinase	Higher in children with Down's syndrome who are more prone to periodontal diseases
Hayakawa et al.1994 [65]	TIMP-1 and total collagenase activity	TIMP-1 was lower in patients with periodontal disease and total collagenase activity was higher in diseased patients

9. Oral cancer and saliva

Oral cancer is 6th most common human malignancies with approximately 50% mortality rate in 5 years. Oral cancer is a potentially lethal disease and the result of the treatment and prognosis largely determined by primary diagnosis. For prevention, treatment and for prognosis, it is essential to measure the disease objectively and accurately in quantitative manner. Quantification of biochemical or molecular specific products of cancers in serum or localised body juices can be one of the current methods of measuring oral cancer objectively. Salivary diagnostics has influenced several researchers and has been verified as an important tool in the diagnosis of many systemic conditions and prognosis of the disease. Developments in the ground of molecular biology, salivary genomics and proteomics have directed to the detection of novel molecular markers for oral cancer diagnosis, therapeutics and prognosis.

Several research groups have found that salivary levels of specific proteins are increased in whole saliva of patients with oral squamous cell carcinoma. For example, CD44 (a cell surface glycoprotein involved in cell-to-cell interaction), 44 Cyfra 21-1 (a fragment of cytokeratin 19), tissue polypeptide antigen (TPS), and cancer antigen 125 (CA-125) have been suggested as oral cancer bio markers [2, 66].

Abundant biomarkers have been studied for finding of oral potentially malignant diseases and cancer, until now no further research has been done. Whole saliva was used to conduct most of the research projects. Whole saliva comprises of juices from all major and minor salivary glands, as well as liquids from mucosal and periodontal tissues, which are influenced by oral and systemic environments and by host immune responses and carry the essence of disease product with them. Measuring the levels of disease product will provide a specific diagnostic and prognostic value. Additionally, least requirement of money, material and manpower makes it more economical, less time consumption, and no special training make this methodology easily accepted.

10. Usage of stimulated or un-stimulated saliva for collection

Unstimulated saliva is considered as an ideal sample because it has no effect on flow rate and salivary composition of salivary glands. But some researches shows that stimulated saliva also can provide equally or more precise detection of cancer biomarkers [67, 68]. Limited researches were performed in these directions on the effect of stimulated and unstimulated saliva on salivary biomarkers of cancer. Hence, it needs to be studied to further standardise the salivary biomarkers.

11. Storage and transportation of saliva

Saliva is very sensitive sample, which is influenced by systemic, physiological, microbial, environmental (food products) and biochemical changes in oral cavity. It also fluctuates with time of collection, Ph of the surrounding environment, temperature type of saliva collection method, and storage methods [69, 70–73] Some study reported that storage at −80°C provides less biochemical and microbial changes in saliva hence gives better results as compared to −20°C [72] . To avoid altered results, there should be least time gap between sample collection and analysis.

12. Classification of salivary biomarkers for oral cancer

Biomarkers have been classified based on biomolecules and disease states [74, 75]. Based on biological molecules:

1. DNA biomarkers

2. RNA biomarkers

3. Protein biomarkers

a. Enzymes

b. Hormones

c. Glycoproteins

4. Salivary ions

5. Oxidative stress assessment

i. Based on disease state

1. Diagnostic biomarkers

2. Prognostic biomarkers

More than 100 potential salivary biomarkers have been reported till date, they can be explained with following headings:

1. Peptides

2. Proteins

3. DNA

4. Salivary mRNA

1. *Peptides*: some of the researches explain that polypeptides like defensin which possess cytotoxic and antimicrobial properties, which exhibits their presence in azurophil granules of polymorphonuclear leukocytes is one of the potent biomarker of oral cancer. OSCC can be distinguished even in their earlier stages by the raised levels of salivary defensin-1 matched with healthy controls [67, 76].

2. *Proteins*: major portion of salivary biomarkers are protein in nature. Most of the proteins share their presence with other diseases or environmental factors (food), this exhibits higher levels of sensitivity with low specificity. Some of the protein biomarkers showed significant elevated level in saliva such as interleukins (8, 6, 1b), matrix metalloproteinase (MMP 2, 9), transforming growth factor (TGF-1), Ki67, cyclic D1, transferrin, amylase, tumour necrosis factor (TNF-a) and catalase among saliva of oral squamous cell carcinoma by various studies [77]. Protein CD44 showed elevated levels in saliva (oral rinse) of oral squamous cell carcinoma patients (n = 102) matched to controls (n = 69) [78]. some of the researches confirmed that IL-8 and IL-6 are informative biomarkers for OSCC, where IL-8 and IL6 showed elevated levels of concentration in saliva and serum respectively [79].

A. Enzymes:

1. *Lysozyme*: lysozyme is an antimicrobial enzyme secreted in human saliva with the capability to hydrolase peptidoglycan, which is the major constituent

of Gram-positive cell wall. Lysozyme shows antitumor properties by direct activation of immune cells or it can raise tumour cell immunogenicity. And also, lysozyme can release elements from bacteria (peptidoglycans and/ or polyribopyrimidinic acids) responsible for immune-potentiation and therefore antitumor activity [80].

2. *Pyruvate kinase M2 isoenzymes*: cancer cell uses metabolic alteration (Warberg's effect) for their survival and growth. They chose anaerobic respiration for their energy needs even though abundant availability of oxygen. Pyruvate kinase muscle iso-enzyme M2 (PKM2) is a glycolytic enzyme and a vital enzyme in tumour cell metabolism and growth. Increased level in serum and saliva indicate presence of malignancy [81].

3. *Collagenase*: collagenase is the major intracellular enzyme explains the destruction of the tissue if found in extracellular fluids like saliva. In saliva this may indicate destruction of periodontal tissue, pulp tissue, infective necrosis or carcinogenic destructions [15].

4. *Acid and alkaline phosphatase*: a study clarifies that the salivary ALP enzyme displays significantly higher levels in subjects with diabetes mellitus, smokers and subjects with potentially malignant disorders without any periodontitis associated to systemically healthy persons [82]

B. Glycoproteins:

Lactic acid and pyruvic acid: pyruvic acid and lactic acids were produced as the end product in the physiologic process of glycolysis [83, 84]. This energy creation cascade carry on by using the end product (pyruvate) of glycolysis as a fuel to Krebs cycle in mitochondria by oxidative phosphorylation. But this process gets interrupted in malignant cells where cell undergoes fermentation of sugar molecule (anaerobic respiration) even though enough presence of oxygen. This process is known as Warberg's effect. This leads to accumulation of the excess PA and LA. Hence quantification can give a clearer picture on the stages of cancer [83].

C. *Salivary ions*: most of the researches explain excess and deficient levels of copper or zinc were significant correlation with oral cancer risk [85]

D. *Oxidative stress assessment*: oxidative stress is the product of a discrepancy between oxidant factors and protective antioxidant systems; it may occur due to an excess of free radicals, or by the shrinking of the antioxidant systems.

Oxidative stress was also associated with oral cancer, as amplified lipid peroxidation and reduced antioxidants was reported in patients suffering from stage II, III, and IV oral cancer [52, 86].

3. *DNA*: DNA is highly specific type of biomarker used for detection of cancer. It requires high end operating machineries and also requires special training to operate it. This makes it more expensive biomarker to detect. Boyle et al. observed that OSCC exhibits p53 mutations in 71% of saliva samples by using plaque hybridization technique [87]. Aberrant methylation of p16, MGMT and DAP-K in OSCC patients was recognised by Rosas et al.

4. *Salivary mRNAs*: oral carcinogenesis can be detected by measuring the elevated six mRNA molecules such as DUSP1, H3F3A, IL 1B, IL 8, SAT and S100 [88].

   a. *DUSP1* (dual specificity phosphatase 1): DUSP mRNA involved in protein modification, oxidative stress, and signal transduction and participates in MAPK (Mitogen Activated Protein Kinase) pathway. Molecular studies showed that the carcinogenesis is associated with hypermethylation of DUSP1 gene [89].

   b. *H3F3A*: these proteins are nuclear proteins, located in chromosome 1, responsible for the structural integrity of chromosomal nucleosome and acts as a one of the proliferative marker for oral cancer.

   c. *IL IB*: Interleukin 1 beta is a chemical mediator of cell proliferation, differentiation, and apoptosis and also inflammation. Though it represents its presence in other pathological and physiological aspects, it shows Elevated serum levels in patients with oral squamous cell carcinoma.

   d. *IL 8*: Interleukin 8 (neutrophil chemotactic factor) is a pro-inflammatory cytokine which plays a key role in tumour angiogenesis, cell adhesion, and cell cycle arrest. By observing various studies on salivary biomarkers, it concluded that IL 8 in saliva is the best biomarker for squamous cell carcinoma [79].

   e. *SAT*: Spermidine/spermine N1-acetyltransferase 1 a protein that participates in the catabolism of polyamines. Researches show elevated levels of SAT in the saliva of oral cancer patients compared to the healthy controls.

   f. *S100 P*: it is a calcium binding protein P, which is located in the cytoplasm or in the nucleus. Its levels in saliva get deviated among oral cancer subjects.

5. *Salivary microRNA*: MicroRNAs (miRNAs) are short parts of RNA transcripts. They are associated with most of the cellular functions like cell growth, apoptosis, differentiation, motility, and immunity. miRNAs are more specific and potent compared to mRNAs. They exhibit high sensitivity which effectively detect and differentiate poorly differentiated carcinomas. Some of these include miR-125a, miR-200a and miR-31 [88].

13. Conclusion

Saliva contains numerous substances which are potential biomarker of many oral diseases. Saliva could be a key cause of biochemical records capable of identifying some diseases. Hence would be useful for ideal methods to diagnosis, prognosis, and monitoring and management of patients with oral diseases. Even though saliva provides some evidence in early detection of oral diseases with advantages like easy, inexpensive, safe, less time and technique sensitive and non-invasive approach over serum, it showed resistance in the diagnostic and clinical usage. Salivary diagnostics faces lots of challenges for the use of saliva-based oral fluid diagnostics for future application. Salivary diagnostic procedures required more sensitive technological support and quality researches to generalise and implement the procedures.

Author details

Manohar Bhat[1]* and Devikripa Bhat[2]

1 Department of Dentistry, Mysore Medical College and Research Institute, Mysore, Karnataka, India

2 Department of Dentistry, S.D.M. College of Dental Sciences and Hospital, Karnataka, India

*Address all correspondence to: manoharpangala@gmail.com

References

[1] Malathi N, Mythili S, Vasanthi HR. Salivary diagnostics: A brief review. ISRN Dentistry. 2014;**2014**:1-8

[2] Javaid MA, Ahmed AS, Durand R, Tran SD. Saliva as a diagnostic tool for oral and systemic diseases. Journal of Oral Biology and Craniofacial Research. 2016;**6**(1):67-76

[3] Mandel ID, Kutscher A, Denning CR, Thompson RH, Zegarelli EV. Salivary studies in cystic fibrosis. American Journal of Diseases of Children. 1967;**113**(4):431-438

[4] Gröschl M. The physiological role of hormones in saliva. BioEssays. 2009;**31**(8):843-852

[5] Pfaffe T, Cooper-White J, Beyerlein P, Kostner K, Punyadeera C. Diagnostic potential of saliva: Current state and future applications. Clinical Chemistry. 2011;**57**(5):675-687

[6] Dowd FJ. Saliva and dental caries. Dental Clinics of North America. 1999;**43**(4):579-597

[7] Peter S. Essentials of Preventive and Community Dentistry (Text Book). Vol. 2. New Delhi: Arya Medi Publishing House; 2004

[8] Siqueira W, Helmerhorst E, Zhang W, Salih E, Oppenheim F. Acquired enamel pellicle and its potential role in oral diagnostics. Annals of the New York Academy of Sciences. 2007;**1098**(1):504-509

[9] Siqueira WL, Oppenheim FG. Small molecular weight proteins/peptides present in the in vivo formed human acquired enamel pellicle. Archives of Oral Biology. 2009;**54**(5):437-444

[10] Vukosavljevic D, Custodio W, Siqueira WL. Salivary proteins as predictors and controls for oral health. Journal of Cell Communication and Signaling. 2011;**5**(4):271-275

[11] Marsh PD. Are dental diseases examples of ecological catastrophes? Microbiology. 2003;**149**(2):279-294

[12] Köhler B, Bratthall D. Practical method to facilitate estimation of *Streptococcus mutans* levels in saliva. Journal of Clinical Microbiology. 1979;**9**(5):584-588

[13] Socransky SS. Caries-susceptibility tests. Annals of the New York Academy of Sciences. 1968;**153**(1):137-146

[14] Güven Y, Satman I, Dinççağ N, Alptekin S. Salivary peroxidase activity in whole saliva of patients with insulin-dependent (type-1) diabetes mellitus. Journal of Clinical Periodontology. 1996;**23**(9):879-881

[15] Hernandez M, Valenzuela MA, Lopez-Otin C, Alvarez J, Lopez JM, Vernal R, et al. Matrix metalloproteinase-13 is highly expressed in destructive periodontal disease activity. Journal of Periodontology. 2006;**77**(11):1863-1870

[16] Dreizen S, Mann AW, Cline J, Spies TD. The buffer capacity of saliva as a measure of dental caries activity. Journal of Dental Research. 1946;**25**(4):213-222

[17] Lenander-Lumikari M, Loimaranta V. Saliva and dental caries. Advances in Dental Research. 2000;**14**(1):40-47

[18] Birkhed D. Salivary secretion rate, buffer capacity, and pH, in human saliva. Clinical Chemistry and Microbiology. 1989;**1**:50-52

[19] Miura H, Isogai E, Hirose K, Wakizaka H, Ueda I, Ito N. Application of a sucrose indicator strip to evaluate salivary sucrose clearance. Journal of Dentistry. 1991;**19**(3):189-191

[20] Van der Reijden W, Van der Kwaak J, Veerman E, Amerongen AN. Analysis of the concentration and output of whole salivary constituents in patients with Sjögren's syndrome. European Journal of Oral Sciences. 1996;**104**(4):335-340

[21] Hadjimarkos D. Effect of selenium on dental caries. Archives of Environmental Health: An International Journal. 1965;**10**(6):893-899

[22] Fox P. Saliva composition and its importance in dental health. Compendium (Newtown, Pa) Supplement. 1989;**13**:S457

[23] Kaufman E, Lamster IB. Analysis of saliva for periodontal diagnosis: A review. Journal of Clinical Periodontology. 2000;**27**(7):453-465

[24] Mandel I, Wotman S. The salivary secretions in health and disease. Oral Sciences Reviews. 1976;**8**:25-47

[25] Mandel ID. The diagnostic uses of saliva. Journal of Oral Pathology and Medicine. 1990;**19**(3):119-125

[26] Edgar W. Saliva: Its secretion, composition and functions. British Dental Journal. 1992;**172**(8):305

[27] Siqueira WL, Dawes C. The salivary proteome: Challenges and perspectives. Proteomics Clinical Applications. 2011;**5**(11-12):575-579

[28] Spielmann N, Wong DT. Saliva: Diagnostics and therapeutic perspectives. Oral Diseases. 2011;**17**(4):345-354

[29] Scannapieco F, Solomon L, Wadenya R. Emergence in human dental plaque and host distribution of amylase-binding streptococci. Journal of Dental Research. 1994;**73**(10):1627-1635

[30] Gibbons R, Etherden I. Fibronectin-degrading enzymes in saliva and their relation to oral cleanliness. Journal of Periodontal Research. 1986;**21**(4):386-395

[31] Oppenheim F, Yang Y-C, Diamond R, Hyslop D, Offner G, Troxler R. The primary structure and functional characterization of the neutral histidine-rich polypeptide from human parotid secretion. The Journal of Biological Chemistry. 1986;**261**(3):1177-1182

[32] Xu T, Levitz S, Diamond R, Oppenheim F. Anticandidal activity of major human salivary histatins. Infection and Immunity. 1991;**59**(8):2549-2554

[33] Jalil R, Ashley F, Wilson R, Wagaiyu E. Concentrations of thiocyanate, hypothiocyanite, 'free' and 'total' lysozyme, lactoferrin and secretory lgA in resting and stimulated whole saliva of children aged 12-14 years and the relationship with plaque accumulation and gingivitis. Journal of Periodontal Research. 1993;**28**(2):130-136

[34] Millan J. Alkaline phosphatases structure, substrate specificity and functional relatedness to other members of a large superfamily of enzymes. Purinergic Signal. 2006;**2**:335-341

[35] Nakamura M, Slots J. Salivary enzymes: Origin and relationship to periodontal disease. Journal of Periodontal Research. 1983;**18**(6):559-569

[36] Nakashima K, Roehrich N, Cimasoni G. Osteocalcin, prostaglandin E2 and alkaline phosphatase in gingival crevicular fluid: Their relations to periodontal status. Journal of Clinical Periodontology. 1994;**21**(5):327-333

[37] Bhat M, Prasad K, Trivedi D, Acharya A. Dental plaque dissolving agents: An in vitro study. International Journal of Advanced Health Sciences. 2014;**1**(3):1-7

[38] Patil PB, Patil BR. Saliva: A diagnostic biomarker of periodontal diseases. Journal of Indian Society of Periodontology. 2011;**15**(4):310

[39] Chrousos GP, Gold PW. The concepts of stress and stress system disorders: Overview of physical and behavioral homeostasis. Journal of the American Medical Association. 1992;**267**(9):1244-1252

[40] Giannobile WV, Beikler T, Kinney JS, Ramseier CA, Morelli T, Wong DT. Saliva as a diagnostic tool for periodontal disease: Current state and future directions. Periodontology 2000. 2009;**50**(1):52-64

[41] Helmerhorst E, Oppenheim F. Saliva: A dynamic proteome. Journal of Dental Research. 2007;**86**(8):680-693

[42] Herr AE, Hatch AV, Throckmorton DJ, Tran HM, Brennan JS, Giannobile WV, et al. Microfluidic immunoassays as rapid saliva-based clinical diagnostics. Proceedings of the National Academy of Sciences. 2007;**104**(13):5268-5273

[43] Syrjänen S, Piironen P, Markkanen H. Free amino-acid composition of wax-stimulated whole saliva in human subjects with healthy periodontium, severe chronic periodontitis and post-juvenile periodontitis. Archives of Oral Biology. 1984;**29**(9):735-738

[44] Syrjänen S, Piironen P, Markkanen H. Free amino-acid content of wax-stimulated human whole saliva as related to periodontal disease. Archives of Oral Biology. 1987;**32**(9):607-610

[45] Delacroix DL, Dive C, Rambaud J, Vaerman J. IgA subclasses in various secretions and in serum. Immunology. 1982;**47**(2):383

[46] Sandholm L, Grönblad E. Salivary immunoglobulins in patients with juvenile periodontitis and their healthy siblings. Journal of Periodontology. 1984;**55**(1):9-12

[47] Klinkhamer JM. Quantitative evaluation of gingivitis and periodontal disease I. The orogranulocytic migratory rate. Periodontics. 1968;**6**(5):207-211

[48] Rindom Schiött C, Löe H. The origin and variation in number of leukocytes in the human saliva. Journal of Periodontal Research. 1970;**5**(1):36-41

[49] Bhadbhade SJ, Acharya AB, Thakur S. Correlation between probing pocket depth and neutrophil counts in dental plaque, saliva, and gingival crevicular fluid. Quintessence International. 2012;**43**(2):111-117

[50] Kanzaki H, Wada S, Narimiya T, Yamaguchi Y, Katsumata Y, Itohiya K, et al. Pathways that regulate ROS scavenging enzymes, and their role in defense against tissue destruction in periodontitis. Frontiers in Physiology. 2017;**8**:351

[51] Kataoka K, Ekuni D, Tomofuji T, Irie K, Kunitomo M, Uchida Y, et al. Visualization of oxidative stress induced by experimental periodontitis in keap1-dependent oxidative stress detector-luciferase mice. International Journal of Molecular Sciences. 2016;**17**(11):1907

[52] Kumar J, Teoh SL, Das S, Mahakknaukrauh P. Oxidative stress in oral diseases: Understanding its relation with other systemic diseases. Frontiers in Physiology. 2017;**8**:693

[53] Ahmadi-Motamayel F, Goodarzi MT, Jamshidi Z, Kebriaei R. Evaluation of salivary and serum antioxidant and oxidative stress statuses in patients with chronic periodontitis: A case-control study. Frontiers in Physiology. 2017;**8**:189

[54] Akalın FA, Baltacıoğlu E, Alver A, Karabulut E. Lipid peroxidation levels and

total oxidant status in serum, saliva and gingival crevicular fluid in patients with chronic periodontitis. Journal of Clinical Periodontology. 2007;**34**(7):558-565

[55] Matthews J, Wright H, Roberts A, Ling-Mountford N, Cooper P, Chapple I. Neutrophil hyper-responsiveness in periodontitis. Journal of Dental Research. 2007;**86**(8):718-722

[56] Pradeep A, Rao NS, Bajaj P, Agarwal E. 8-Isoprostane: A lipid peroxidation product in gingival crevicular fluid in healthy, gingivitis and chronic periodontitis subjects. Archives of Oral Biology. 2013;**58**(5):500-504

[57] Socransky S, Haffajee A, Cugini M, Smith C, Kent R Jr. Microbial complexes in subgingival plaque. Journal of Clinical Periodontology. 1998;**25**(2):134-144

[58] Zambon JJ, Nakamura M, Slots J. Effect of periodontal therapy on salivary enzymatic activity. Journal of Periodontal Research. 1985;**20**(6):652-659

[59] Gregory R, Kim D, Kindle J, Hobbs L, Lloyd D. Immunoglobulin-degrading enzymes in localized juvenile periodontitis. Journal of Periodontal Research. 1992;**27**(3):176-183

[60] Nieminen A, Nordlund L, Uitto VJ. The effect of treatment on the activity of salivary proteases and glycosidases in adults with advanced periodontitis. Journal of Periodontology. 1993;**64**(4):297-301

[61] Ingman T, Sorsa T, Lindy O, Koski H, Konttinen YT. Multiple forms of gelatinases/type IV collagenases in saliva and gingival crevicular fluid of periodontitis patients. Journal of Clinical Periodontology. 1994;**21**(1):26-31

[62] Uitto VJ, Suomalainen K, Sorsa T. Salivary collagenase. Origin, characteristics and relationship to periodontal health. Journal of Periodontal Research. 1990;**25**(3):135-142

[63] Orner G. Periodontal disease among children with Down's syndrome and their siblings. Journal of Dental Research. 1976;**55**(5):778-782

[64] Halinen S, Sorsa T, Ding Y, Ingman T, Salo T, Konttinen YT, et al. Characterization of matrix metalloproteinase (MMP-8 and-9) activities in the saliva and in gingival crevicular fluid of children with Down's syndrome. Journal of Periodontology. 1996;**67**(8):748-754

[65] Hayakawa H, Yamashita K, Ohwaki K, Sawa M, Noguchi T, Iwata K, et al. Collagenase activity and tissue inhibitor of metalloproteinases-1 (TIMP-1) content in human whole saliva from clinically healthy and periodontally diseased subjects. Journal of Periodontal Research. 1994;**29**(5):305-308

[66] Nagler R, Bahar G, Shpitzer T, Feinmesser R. Concomitant analysis of salivary tumor markers—A new diagnostic tool for oral cancer. Clinical Cancer Research. 2006;**12**(13):3979-3984

[67] Kaur J, Jacobs R, Huang Y, Salvo N, Politis C. Salivary biomarkers for oral cancer and pre-cancer screening: A review. Clinical Oral Investigations. 2018:1-8

[68] Streckfus CF, Dubinsky WP. Proteomic analysis of saliva for cancer diagnosis. Expert Review of Proteomics. 2007;**4**(3):329-332

[69] Nobbs A, Jenkinson H, Jakubovics N. Critical reviews in Oral Biology & Medicine. Journal of Dental Research. 2011;**90**(11):1271-1278

[70] Caporossi L, Santoro A, Papaleo B. Saliva as an analytical matrix: State of the

art and application for biomonitoring. Biomarkers. 2010;**15**(6):475-487

[71] Mohamed R, Campbell J-L, Cooper-White J, Dimeski G, Punyadeera C. The impact of saliva collection and processing methods on CRP, IgE, and myoglobin immunoassays. Clinical and Translational Medicine. 2012;**1**(1):19

[72] Schipper R, Loof A, De Groot J, Harthoorn L, Van Heerde W, Dransfield E. Salivary protein/peptide profiling with SELDI-TOF-MS. Annals of the New York Academy of Sciences. 2007, 1098;(1):498-503

[73] Al-Tarawneh SK, Border MB, Dibble CF, Bencharit S. Defining salivary biomarkers using mass spectrometry-based proteomics: A systematic review. Omics: A Journal of Integrative Biology. 2011;**15**(6):353-361

[74] Radhika T, Jeddy N, Nithya S, Muthumeenakshi R. Salivary biomarkers in oral squamous cell carcinoma—An insight. Journal of Oral Biology and Craniofacial Research. 2016;**6**:S51-SS4

[75] Mishra A, Verma M. Cancer biomarkers: Are we ready for the prime time? Cancers. 2010;**2**(1):190-208

[76] Mizukawa N, Sugiyama K, Fukunaga J, Ueno T, Mishima K, Takagi S, et al. Defensin-1, a peptide detected in the saliva of oral squamous cell carcinoma patients. Anticancer Research. 1998;**18**(6B):4645-4649

[77] Nagler RM, Barak M, Peled M, Ben-Aryeh H, Filatov M, Laufer D. Early diagnosis and treatment monitoring roles of tumor markers Cyfra 21-1 and TPS in oral squamous cell carcinoma. Cancer. 1999;**85**(5):1018-1025

[78] Franzmann EJ, Reategui EP, Pedroso F, Pernas FG, Karakullukcu BM, Carraway KL, et al. Soluble CD44 is a potential marker for the early detection of head and neck cancer. Cancer Epidemiology and Prevention Biomarkers. 2007;**16**(7):1348-1355

[79] MAS J, Li Y, Zhou X, Denny P, Ho C-M, Montemagno C, et al. Interleukin 6 and interleukin 8 as potential biomarkers for oral cavity and oropharyngeal squamous cell carcinoma. Archives of otolaryngology—Head & Neck Surgery. 2004;**130**(8):929-935

[80] Sava G, Benetti A, Ceschia V, Pacor S. Lysozyme and cancer: Role of exogenous lysozyme as anticancer agent. Anticancer Research. 1989;**9**(3):583-591

[81] Dong G, Mao Q, Xia W, Xu Y, Wang J, Xu L, et al. PKM2 and cancer: The function of PKM2 beyond glycolysis. Oncology Letters. 2016;**11**(3):1980-1986

[82] Prakash AR, Indupuru K, Sreenath G, Kanth MR, AVS R, Indira Y. Salivary alkaline phosphatase levels speak about association of smoking, diabetes and potentially malignant diseases??? Journal of Oral and Maxillofacial Pathology. 2016;**20**(1):66

[83] Bhat MA, Prasad K, Trivedi D, Rajeev B, Battur H. Pyruvic acid levels in serum and saliva: A new course for oral cancer screening? Journal of Oral and Maxillofacial Pathology. 2016;**20**(1):102

[84] Nelson DL, Lehninger AL, Cox MM. Lehninger Principles of Biochemistry. New York: Macmillan; 2008

[85] Chen F, Wang J, Chen J, Yan L, Hu Z, Wu J, et al. Serum copper and zinc levels and the risk of oral cancer: A new insight based on large-scale case–control study. Oral Diseases. 2019;**25**(1):80-86

[86] Manoharan S, Kolanjiappan K, Suresh K, Panjamurthy K. Lipid

peroxidation & antioxidants status in patients with oral squamous cell carcinoma. The Indian Journal of Medical Research. 2005;**122**(6):529

[87] Boyle P, Levin B. World Cancer Report 2008. IARC Press, International Agency for Research on Cancer; 2008

[88] Liu J, Duan Y. Saliva: A potential media for disease diagnostics and monitoring. Oral Oncology. 2012;**48**(7):569-577

[89] Khor GH, Froemming GRA, Zain RB, Abraham MT, Omar E, Tan SK, et al. DNA methylation profiling revealed promoter hypermethylation-induced silencing of p16, DDAH2 and DUSP1 in primary oral squamous cell carcinoma. International Journal of Medical Sciences. 2013;**10**(12):1727

Chapter 5

Salivary Biomarkers to Assess Breast Cancer Diagnosis and Progression: Are We There Yet?

Charles F. Streckfus

Abstract

Technological developments are propelling medical diagnostics forward at unprecedented rates. Advancements in genomic, proteomics and cellomics are leading the way for diagnostic tests that will be capable of rapid multi-analyte detection in both laboratory and non-laboratory settings. Currently, proof-of-principle has been demonstrated for salivary biomarkers, whose up and down regulation has been shown to correlate strongly with breast cancer among women. Consequently, the rationale for this chapter is to review the medical literature and present the current research focused on the use of saliva as a diagnostic medium for the study of early breast cancer progression.

Keywords: breast cancer progression, saliva, cancer proteomics, breast cancer, omics, cancer detection, Her2/neu, mass spectrometry, cancer molecular pathways

1. Introduction

Reducing the overall morbidity and mortality rates for carcinoma of the breast is the overall goal of the Department of Health and Human Services [1]. As stated in *Healthy People 2020*, breast cancer is the second leading cause of death in women in the United States, with over 45,000 women dying from the disease each year. Additionally, in the United States, in 2019, it is estimated that 268,600 women and 2670 men will be diagnosed with invasive breast cancer. Additionally, another 62,930 women will be diagnosed with in situ breast cancer [2–7].

Taken together, the chances of a woman being diagnosed with breast cancer during her lifetime have increased. In 1975, the rate was 1 in 11; whereupon today the rate is roughly 1 in 8 [2]. Overall, the number of women being diagnosed continues to increase. This is due in part to the increase in the number of women in age groups at risk of breast cancer. Currently, the median age at which breast cancer is diagnosed is 62 [4–7].

There is also an increase in breast cancer screening which has resulted in a dramatic increase in the incidence of ductal carcinoma in situ (DCIS). DCIS is an early stage, pre-invasive form of breast cancer with a cause-specific survival rate of approximately 100%. The current problem, however, is that it is not possible to distinguish DCIS that will develop into invasive cancer. Consequently, the overdiagnosis and overtreatment of DCIS remains a persistent problem [8, 9].

While breast cancer screening with mammography has been shown in randomized controlled trials to reduce breast cancer-specific mortality, there remains ongoing controversy regarding the value of mammography and its utilization.

Additionally, studies using mathematical modeling suggest that more frequent mammographic screening would further increase patient survival. Analysis of these data suggests a 96% survival rate if patients could receive a mammogram every 3 months. However, due to the costs coupled with the invasiveness of the procedure, this increase in the frequency of mammography is currently not feasible [10].

While advances in imaging have increased breast cancer detectability there are still overarching challenges that need to be addressed. The FY19 BCRP funding announcement succinctly outlines these challenges [11]: (1) prevent breast cancer, (2) identify determinants of breast cancer initiation, risk, or susceptibility, (3) distinguish deadly from non-deadly breast cancers, (4) address the problems of over-diagnosis and overtreatment, (5) identify what drives breast cancer growth; and determine how to stop it, (6) identify why some breast cancers become metastatic, (7) determine why/how breast cancer cells lie dormant for years and then re-emerge, (8) determine how to prevent lethal recurrence, (9) revolutionize treatment regimens by replacing them with ones that are more effective, less toxic, and impact survival, and (10) eliminate the mortality associated with metastatic cancer [11, 12].

The author would like to add two more items: (1) ascertain methods to determine the efficacy of treatment and (2) ascertain methods to determine that the treated patient is not only in *clinical remission*, but in *molecular remission* as well [13, 14]. The latter action items would assure successful treatment.

Taken together, there remains a necessity to identify novel approaches that improve breast cancer screening and early detection. This, in turn, reduces the problems of over-diagnosis and over-treatment and can detect cancers at a point where interventions maybe more effective [1–14].

2. Significant single analyte salivary biomarker studies

There is a paucity of studies in the medical literature concerning the use of saliva for the detection of breast cancer. These reports deal primarily with the identification and quantification of cancer-related proteins, in saliva that were previously discovered to be present in serum or cancer tissue supernatants of diagnosed cancer patients. The importance of these studies establishes the basic groundwork and feasibility of salivary cancer diagnostics and ascertains the basis for continued biomarker research [15].

2.1 Kallikrein

A study that serves to establish the basis for salivary cancer biomarker research methodology comes from a report of kallikrein being used as a diagnostic marker. The investigation reports the use of saliva to detect variations in the concentrations of kallikrein, a regulatory protease, among healthy individuals and patients with malignant breast and gastro-intestinal tumors. The outcome of their investigation revealed elevated concentrations of salivary kallikrein among individuals diagnosed with malignant tumors in comparison with those individuals diagnosed with benign tumors and those from a healthy cohort. Kallikrein was measured by chromogenic tripeptide assay [16].

2.2 Epidermal growth factor

Epidermal growth factor (EGF) is a regulatory growth factor protein responsible for tissue growth and repair [17]. Since EGF overexpression is implicated in tumorigenesis, it may therefore be useful as a tumor marker. Based on this thinking, an additional study [17] demonstrated that EGF concentrations were higher in the saliva of women with primary or recurrent breast cancer in comparison with women lacking a malignancy [17]. The highest concentrations of EGF were found in the local recurrence subgroup, suggesting a potential use for this marker in the post-operative follow-up of diagnosed cancer patients [18].

2.3 The Her2/neu studies

Salivary Her2/neu (e-*erb*B-2) is probably the most thoroughly investigated biomarker [19–21] that is still under current investigation [22–24]. The original investigators [19–21] selected the salivary protein as the biomarker of choice, because this protein was previously shown to be immunohistologically present on the membrane of the ductal epithelium of salivary gland tissues [25, 26]. Additionally, Her2/neu was found in serum [27] and, therefore, provided the investigators with a basis for analytical humoral comparison [28]. Collectively, these points provided the basis for the selection of Her2/neu as a salivary biomarker. CA 15-3 was the gold standard for comparison in both the saliva and serum specimens [19–21].

The results of these studies demonstrated elevated concentrations of the Her2/neu and CA 15-3 proteins in the saliva and serum of all three groups of women. The salivary and serological levels of Her2/neu among the cancer patients were significantly higher ($p < 0.001$) than the salivary and serum levels of healthy controls and benign tumor patients. Additionally, the Her2/neu protein was found to be equal to or to surpass the ability of CA 15-3 to detect cancer patients. The sensitivity and specificity were 87 and 65%, respectively, with a cut-point of 100 Units/ml. These results were comparable with the serum levels of Her2/neu [19–21]. Tumor staging and receptor status were also assessed. Her2/neu increased with staging, but not with Her2/neu status. The finding was later supported by other researchers [23, 29].

Concurrent with the aforementioned investigation, studies to determine the relationship between Her2/neu protein concentrations and various demographic and clinical variables we conducted. These variables potentially could confound the results of any salivary biomarker research. Consequently, the effects of race, age, weight, BMI, tobacco usage, alcohol consumption systemic illnesses (e.g., diabetes, hypertension, etc.), the use of prescription medications, hormonal status and estrogen usage [30], salivary flow rates, marker contributions from epithelia present in saliva, and the presence of periodontal disease on salivary Her2/neu concentrations were assessed. Edentulous patients were also assessed to control for the effects of periodontal disease. These studies show that these potentially confounding variables exact no effect on salivary Her2/neu concentrations [19–21].

Two other questions that needed to be answered are as follows: could the pungent chemotherapeutics used in cancer treatment adversely affect Her2/neu salivary concentrations and secondly could tumor removal and post-chemotherapy events modulate, in this case lower, salivary Her2/neu concentrations. In response, a study was conducted to answer the aforementioned questions and to establish the utility of the salivary Her2/neu in monitoring patients diagnosed with carcinoma of the breast before and after treatment.

Twenty-five patients with various stages of carcinoma of the breast were followed through the course of treatment. ELISA assays for Her2/neu and CA 15-3 were performed on their serum and stimulated whole-saliva specimens. These baseline samples were collected from all patients prior to the administration of any adjunct therapy or surgery and were sequentially sampled during therapy and after their treatment. As noted in **Figure 1**, the outcome of the study demonstrated the modulation of Her2/neu concentrations in response to chemotherapeutic treatment. Additionally, it may be useful to detect post-treatment recurrence. Indeed, salivary Her2/neu may have the potential to track treatment success and guide therapy. The salivary Her2/neu determinations also mirrored those for serum Her2/neu and CA 15-3 [31].

Finally, a clinical experiment was conducted to ascertain the reliability and repeatability of detecting Her2/neu in both 9 healthy men and 10 healthy women over a 5-day time-period [32]. The individuals were saliva sampled at 9 AM., 4 PM. and 9 PM. over the 5-day period. The samples were stored at −80°C and later assayed by ELISA for the Her2/neu protein. The results exhibited no demonstrable salivary Her2/neu differences regarding gender, day or time of collection. Inter and intra correlation coefficients did decrease in the 4 PM. and 9 PM. collections suggesting that morning to afternoon collections may be optimal for collecting salivary Her2/neu specimens [32].

2.3.1 Other supporting experiments

Other technologies were employed to support the aforementioned clinical findings [32]. Using Her2/neu antibodies, the authors executed several Western blot experiments. The first of these experiments compared saliva and serum concentrations of Her2/neu in specimens from among seven healthy subjects. The blot demonstrated protein presence at a range of 170–185 kDa, with denser bands being revealed in the salivary samples. A second Western blot to ascertain which salivary gland(s) were producing the salivary Her2/neu. Saliva collected from the parotid and submandibular glands, and total whole saliva, were sampled from two healthy individuals. The results

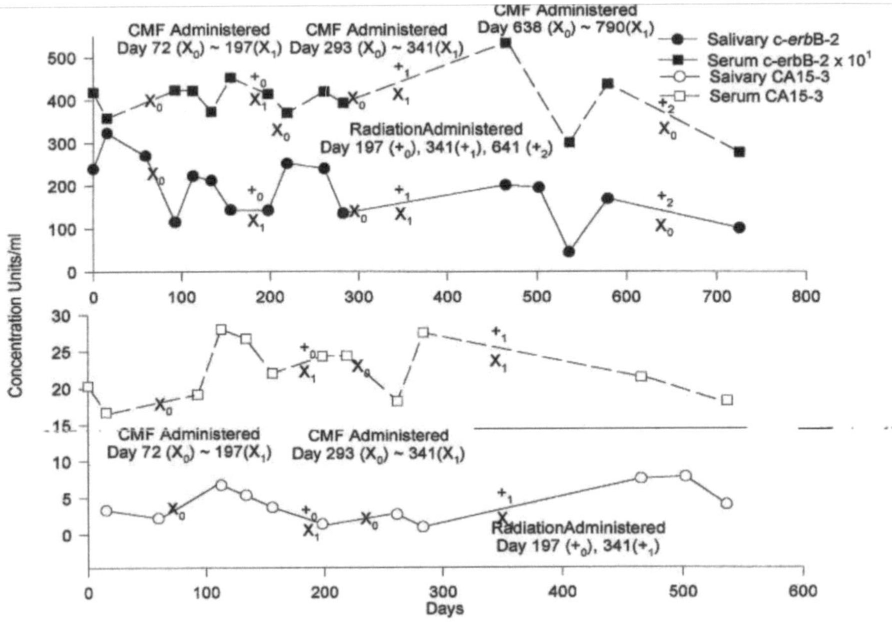

Figure 1.
An example of post-operative monitoring. The upper graph represents salivary and serum c-erbB-2 concentrations across time of treatment. The lower graph represents salivary and serum CA 15-3 concentrations across time of treatment. As illustrated, the c-erbB-2 concentrations are in concordance with the commonly used CA 15-3 cancer biomarker [31].

suggest that all the major salivary glands were contributors of Her2/neu salivary secretions regardless if the glands were serous (parotid) or mixed (submandibular) saliva producers. A third experiment compared Her2/neu salivary secretions between three individuals diagnosed with carcinoma of the breast and two healthy controls. The Western blot demonstrated denser 170–185-kDa bands among the cancer subjects as compared with healthy controls. The conclusions derived from these experiments suggest that Her2/neu is increased in saliva secondary to carcinoma of the breast [33].

An animal study was also conducted determine if Her2/neu can be detected from a remote areas of the body [34]. Male rat saliva does not contain salivary Her2/neu. Consequently, two male Sprague-Dawley rats, each weighing between 300 and 500 g, were used. One experimental animal received 200 μl, and the other, 500 μl, of encapsulated Her2/neu protein. The capsulated Her2/neu proteins were placed in the peritoneum of each rat. Prior to capsule placement, baseline serum and saliva samples were taken. Samples were also taken 20, 68, 140, 188, 308 and 356 hours post-placement. Saliva flow was induced by administration of ophthalmic pilocarpine prior to sampling. All samples were kept at −20°C. Antibody detection was performed using a modified double capture ELISA system. The animal receiving the higher antibody concentration showed a markedly greater salivary level of the antibody than the other (peak 24.158 vs. 18.313 HNU/ml at 308 and 188 hours post-implantation, respectively). Baseline values were below detection for both animals. These results appear to indicate that Her2/neu may be detected from remote areas of the body [34].

A different type of platform, surface-enhanced laser desorption/ionization mass spectrometry (SELDI), was employed to confirm the presence and alteration of Her2/neu in saliva [35]. The results of the preliminary SELDI assays were encouraging. The weak cation exchange (WCX @ pH 3.5) biochip demonstrated the most potential for profiling salivary proteins. Interestingly, a protein cluster in the range of 170 kDa (**Figure 2**) was more prevalent in cancer patient saliva samples than in

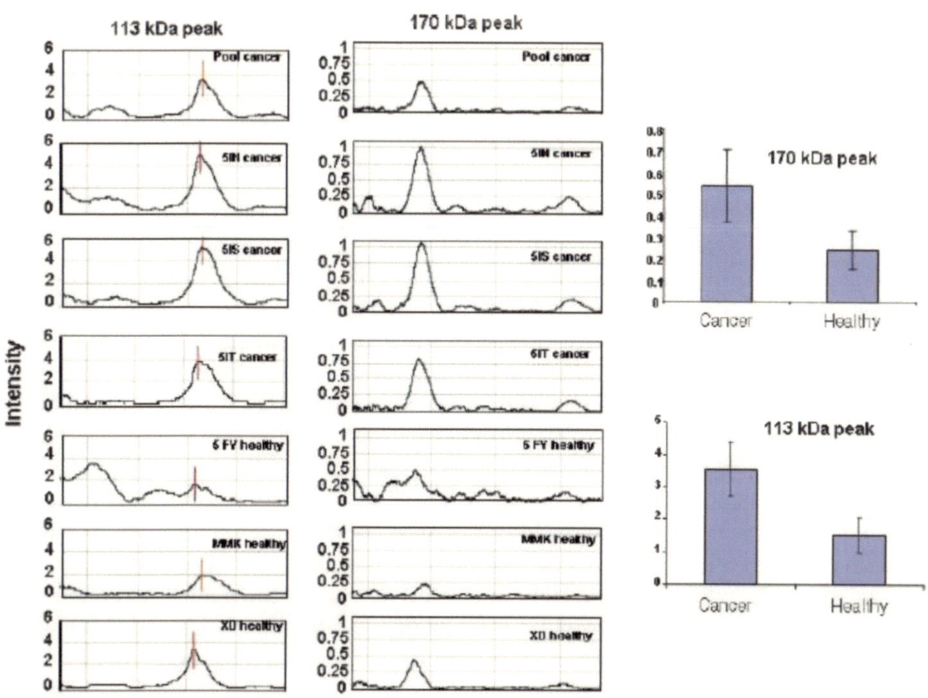

Figure 2.
The 113 and 117 kDa spectral peaks in saliva. Additionally, bar graphs to the right show mean values for the 113 and 117 kDa spectral peaks [35].

samples from normal subjects [36]. Also of note, one of the donors in the normal group (XD) is known by ELISA to have quite high Her2/neu levels and stands out from the other two normal donors in this analysis. These similar results were also demonstrated by serum and the extract from the SKBR-3 breast cancer cell lines with SELDI analyses.

In addition, an increase of the proteins in this range from cancer patient saliva, especially in the range of approximately 113 kDa, can be seen in **Figure 2**. One possible cancer-related biomarker is the extracellular domain (ECD) of Her2/neu receptor, which is approximately 110 kDa (deglycosylated), based on two-dimensional and Western blot gel analyses.

3. Proteomics studies for salivary biomarkers and their findings

Mass spectrometry and liquid chromatography have enabled the researchers to analyze complex peptide mixtures with the ability to detect proteins differing in abundance by over eight orders of magnitude. Isotopic labeling coupled with liquid chromatography tandem mass spectrometry (IL-LC-MS/MS) is often used to characterize the salivary proteome. The approach readily identifies changes in the level of expression, thus permitting the analysis of putative regulatory pathways providing information regarding the pathological disturbances in addition to potential biomarkers of disease.

A PubMed.gov database search yielded a paucity of manuscripts (15) using LC/MS/MS mass spectrometry. The majority of the manuscripts were composed by the author of this chapter [37–40]. In these manuscripts, the researchers used an Applied Biosystems QStar® XL LC/MS/MS mass spectrometer equipped with an LC Packings high performance liquid chromatography (HPLC) for capillary chromatography. The HPLC was coupled to the mass spectrometer by a nanospray ESI head for maximal sensitivity. The advantage of tandem mass spectrometry combined with LC is enhanced sensitivity and the peptide separations afforded by chromatography. Thus even in complex protein mixtures MS/MS data can be used to sequence and identify peptides either by peptide similarity or sequence analysis with a high degree of confidence [41–44].

The researchers employed iTRAQ reagents [37–39] that are amino reactive compounds. The real advantage of using iTRAQ is that the tags remain intact through TOF MS analysis. This in turn enables the tags to be revealed during collision-induced dissociation by MS/MS analysis. Thus in the MS/MS spectrum for each peptide, there is a pattern indicating the quantity of that peptide from each of the different protein pools. Essentially all of the peptides in a mixture are labeled by the reaction; numerous proteins are identified and can be compared for their relative concentrations in each mixture. Thus, even in complex mixtures there is a high degree of confidence in the identification because of the large number of peptides that can be used for protein identification.

Pooled samples were used in these studies with full knowledge of the advantages and shortcomings for the technique [45]. Considering that, the exploratory findings would have to be validated using other laboratory methodologies, the researchers decided to use the pooled sample technique. Sample size for the pooled specimens was also calculated [45]. The sample size for each pool was 10 subjects. Additionally, the authors used a *positive control* (benign tumors), which is not found in many of the breast cancer biomarker experiments using saliva as the diagnostic media. To enhance the study, the same samples were assayed by a *blinded outside laboratory* [37].

Using the LC-MS/MS platform, the researchers used a three-prong approach to obtain salivary protein profiles of cancer patients. The first was to determine if the technology could detect the smallest ductal carcinoma lesions (Stage 0, Stage I) and compare their profiles to those of a positive control (fibroadenomas) and healthy individuals [37]. The second parameter was to determine protein profile differences between lymph node positive and lymph node negative cancer patients [38]. Third experiment was to ascertain differences between Her2/neu receptor positive and Her2/neu receptor negative individuals [39]. Taken together, these three major parameters influence tumor progression.

The initial study compared the protein profiles of four cohorts: healthy, benign tumor, Stage 0 and Stage I [37]. The PathwayStudio® software, a bioinformatics software package was used to determine the fold increase/decrease and p-values. p-Values equal to or less than 0.001 were used to select the best biomarker candidates. The number of proteins for each group is shown in **Table 1**.

The panel (**Table 1**) has putative markers that are both up and/or down regulated and have varying cellular functions. These proteins are validated in cell studies and found altered in the presence of carcinoma of the breast.

The aim of the second study was to compare the salivary protein profiles of pooled saliva specimens from individuals diagnosed with ductal carcinoma of the breast

Comparison	Upregulated	Downregulated	Total markers
Healthy vs. benign	19	10	29
Healthy vs. Stage 0	15	15	30
Healthy vs. Stage I	9	17	26
Benign vs. cancers	9	6	15

Table 1.
The up- and downregulated proteins for each cohort.

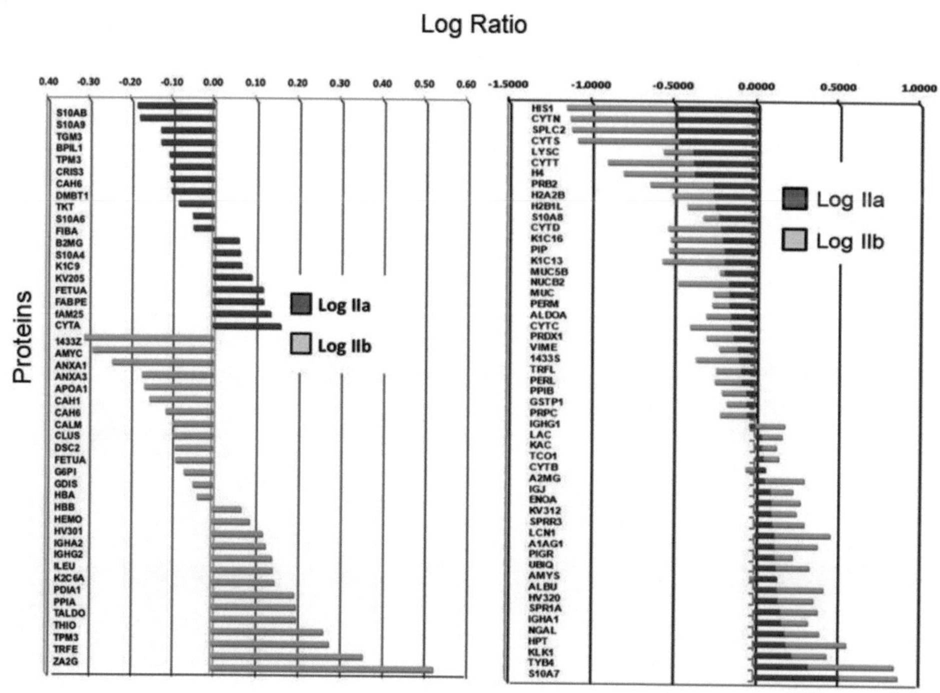

Figure 3.
The differential expression of salivary proteins common and different to both Stage IIa and Stage IIb [38].

with and without lymph node involvement [38]. Three pooled (n = 10 subjects/pooled specimen) stimulated whole saliva specimens from women were analyzed. One pooled specimen was from healthy women, another pooled specimen was from women diagnosed with Stage IIa ($T_2N_0M_0$) invasive ductal carcinoma (IDC) without lymph node involvement and one pooled specimen was from women diagnosed with Stage IIb ($T_2N_1M_0$) with lymph node involvement. Experimentally, saliva from each of the pooled samples was trypsinized and the peptide digests labeled with the appropriate iTRAQ reagent. The results are shown in **Figure 3**. The analyses yielded approximately 174 differentially expressed proteins in the saliva specimens. Fifty-five proteins were common to both cancer stages while there were there were 20 proteins unique to Stage IIa and 28 proteins that were unique to Stage IIb. The proteins are listed in **Figure 3**. The study suggests that salivary proteomic profiles may be useful in determining lymph node involvement among cancer patients [38].

The third aspect was to compare the salivary profiles from subjects diagnosed with breast cancer that were either Her2/neu receptor positive or negative. As previously mentioned, two pooled saliva specimens underwent proteomic analysis. One pooled specimen was from women diagnosed with Stage IIa, Her2/neu receptor positive breast cancer patients (n = 10) and the other was from women diagnosed with Stage IIb, Her2/neu receptor negative (n = 10). The pooled samples were trypsinized and the peptides labeled with iTRAQ reagent. Specimens were analyzed using a LC-MS/MS mass spectrometer. The results yielded approximately 71 differentially expressed proteins in the saliva specimens. There were 34 up-regulated proteins and 37 down regulated proteins. **Figure 4** provides a visualization of the saliva protein differences between positive and negative Her2/neu receptor status [39].

Validation of the makers resulting from these studies was performed in a number of studies [46–49]. The results of all these studies plus numerous others were finally comprised into a manuscript, which presents a *catalogue of salivary proteins* that have been altered in the presence of ductal carcinoma of the breast. These findings are supported by other proteomic analysis of breast cancer cell lines, breast cancer tissues, tissue microenvironment and serum [40]. Additionally, nearly 29% of the panel of proteins has been technically validated by either Western blot or by ELISA. A breakdown of these proteins has also been analyzed according staging and Her2/neu receptor status. All of the proteins were sorted according to their *function*. A *pathway analysis* was also employed. The investigators have also found that the protein concentrations can be modulated while undergoing cancer treatment and respond differently according pathological cell type [40].

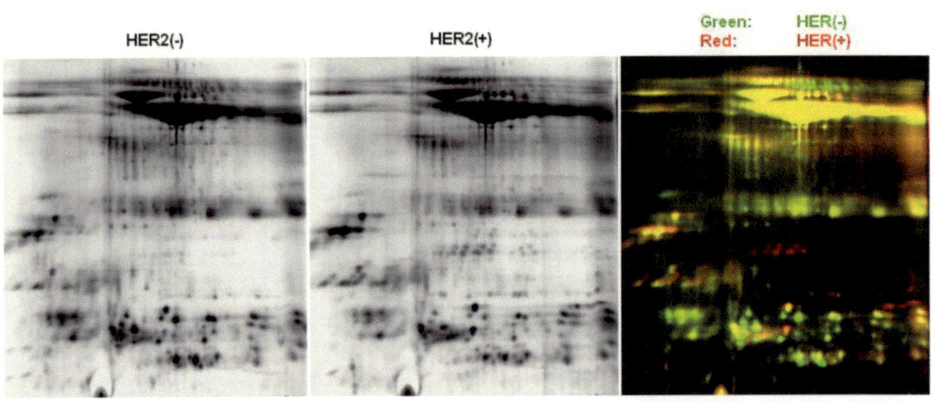

Figure 4.
The protein profiles for HER2/neu receptor positive and HER2/neu receptor negative samples. As shown in the far right red and green dyed gel comparisons, there are numerous differences between the two profiles [39].

One major result of these and other studies is the standardization of saliva collection and preparation for storage [50]. Additionally, standards for proteomic analysis have been established [51].

4. Salivary transcriptome: mRNA and miRNA

In a number of studies conducted by Wong et al., they discovered the presence and utility of mRNA in saliva for the detection of breast cancer [52–55]. These findings not only provided researchers with a new source of biomarkers, but also a new method for cross-validating proteomic findings [55]. Taken together, these studies helped explain preexisting studies and further served to illustrate the complexity of salivary composition [52–55].

Concurrent with these studies, were investigations assessing salivary miRNA as potential biomarkers for breast cancer detection [56, 57]. These studies also demonstrated how gene microarray and quantitative real-time PCR technology, could detect micro-RNA candidates [56, 57]. It has been demonstrated that, secondary to breast cancer, salivary micro-RNA profiles are altered [56, 57].

5. Salivary exosomes and microvesicles

One of the major questions regarding salivary biomarker research is how large proteins, mRNA and miRNA enter the saliva proper. Many proteins are too large to pass through the intercellular spaces of the acinar cells. So how do they enter whole saliva? Additionally, RNAs are intracellular proteins making the problem even more complex.

In 2012, Lau and Wong demonstrated how these particulates might enter the saliva via *exosome—like microvesicles* [58]. The investigators employed an *in vitro* breast cancer model that demonstrated that breast cancer derived exosome—like

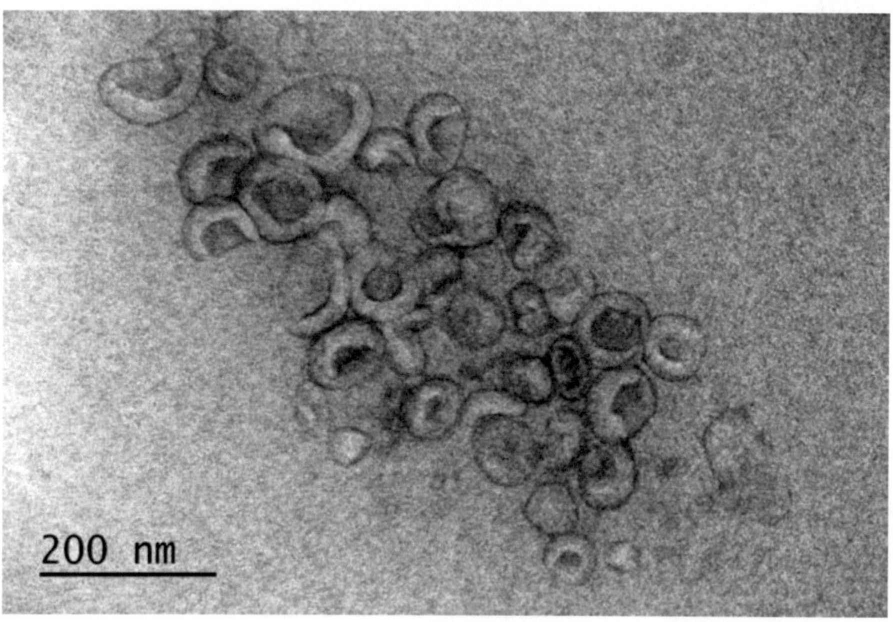

Figure 5.
An electron micrograph of extracellular vesicles (courtesy of Maija Puhka, Ph.D. of the EV CORE and Institute for Molecular Medicine Finland FIMM, University of Helsinki, Finland).

microvesicles interact with salivary gland cells and produce an altered salivary profile. Within these exosome—like microvesicles they found proteins and mRNA. They also found that the exosome—like microvesicles communicated and activated the transcriptional activity of the salivary glands. The result of this activity altered the composition of salivary gland exosome—like microvesicles and the ensuing salivary secretion [58].

Subsequent research has yielded numerous vesicular structures, which can bind to a suitable receptor on a target cell [59–61]. These bodies include exosomes, ectosomes, apoptotic bodies and extracellular vesicles (**Figure 5**). Once thought to be repositories for cellular waste, these vesicular bodies provide intricate functions in intercellular communication and compound exchange. Current research is demonstrating that these vesicular bodies mediate disease progression. Subsequent research has shown this finding to be of great utility in under-standing altered salivary composition secondary to various disease states [59–61].

It is also worth noting that extracellular vesicles may also explain the findings reported in Section 2.2 of this chapter as Andre et al. extracted Her2/neu from exosomal pellets [62]. This may be the underlying mechanism by which biomarker proteins enter saliva.

6. Metabolites

In a study conducted by Sugimoto et al., the investigators assessed the diagnostic utility *metabolites* in saliva [63]. They conducted a comprehensive metabolite analysis of saliva samples obtained from 215 individuals. Sixty-nine subjects were diagnosed with oral cancer, 18 with pancreatic cancer and 30 with carcinoma of the breast. These cohorts were compared to 11 periodontal disease patients and 87 healthy controls. They used capillary electrophoresis time-of-flight mass spectrometry (CE-TOF-MS). Fifty-seven principal metabolites were identified that accurately predicted the probability of being affected by each individual disease. Additionally they were found that between the known patient characteristics and the quantified metabolites, the profiles manifested relatively higher concentrations in most of the metabolites in all three cancers as compared to those in people with periodontal disease and control subjects. Several metabolites in breast cancer patients yielded a statistically significant difference between breast cancer and healthy controls, including taurine and lysine. However, there were no differences in metabolites between breast cancer and other two cancers. These metabolites are promising biomarkers for cancer screening [63, 64].

7. Conclusions

Based on the volume of evidence provided in this review, the author believes that that saliva may have diagnostic potential and the potential to be used to study breast cancer progression. As described throughout this text, different analytes using various biochemical platforms have all indicated that the constituents in saliva are altered secondary to breast cancer. The logistic utility of this media has been described in numerous manuscripts; however, to date there are no FDA approved salivary diagnostic devices for the detection of breast on the commercial market despite the fact that many of these findings have been patented.

Considering the logistical advantages of salivary diagnostic testing and the deadliness of the disease we are trying to detect, it would be extremely useful to continue to explore the possibility of using saliva as a medium for treatment efficacy and tumor recurrence. Post-treatment monitoring for breast cancer recurrence is extremely important. The patient may be in *clinical remission* but not necessarily in *molecular remission* [40, 65]. This could be accomplished using a microarray containing salivary marker of the varying cancer pathways associated with carcinoma of the breast [40]. Post-treatment serial sampling would indicate the efficacy and indicate protein changes, which could lead to tumor recurrence.

Besides commercialization, Karachi et al. (1985) presented a lingering problem to the salivary research community [65]. While at N.I.H., he conducted an experiment whereby he removed the submandibular gland of virgin mice 14–22 weeks old. This resulted in a reduced the tumor incidence to 12.8% (n = 39) at the age of 52 weeks and also increased the latency period of mammary tumor development as much as 14 weeks when compared to that of normal mice. Long-term treatment of sialoadenectomized virgin mice with EGF increased the tumor incidence to 33.3%. Moreover, sialoadenectomy of mammary tumor-bearing animals caused a rapid and sustained cessation of tumor growth, but EGF administration quickly restored the rate of tumor growth to a normal level. These results indicate that submandibular gland EGF plays a crucial role in mouse mammary tumorigenesis [65].

The aforementioned study suggests an influence of salivary EGF on tumorigenesis. Additionally, it is known from other salivary studies that EGF is elevated in human saliva secondary to breast cancer [17, 18]. Could the same effect mentioned by Karachi be taking place in humans? [65].

In addition, another study reported an increase in salivary protein rich peptides levels among breast cancer patients [40, 48]. Using a proline rich peptide segment (p1978) from the parent SMR3B protein peptide in saliva, the researchers found that this peptide inhibited the growth of HCC38 triple-negative cancer cells [48]. Perhaps the elevation of in of this peptide is in response to tumor proliferation. It is known that proline-rich-peptides have a high affinity to the Grb2/SH3 domain, which in turn inhibits Ras activation by blocking Sos binding to Grb2 receptor. Taken together both studies suggest feedback systems as illustrated in **Figure 6**.

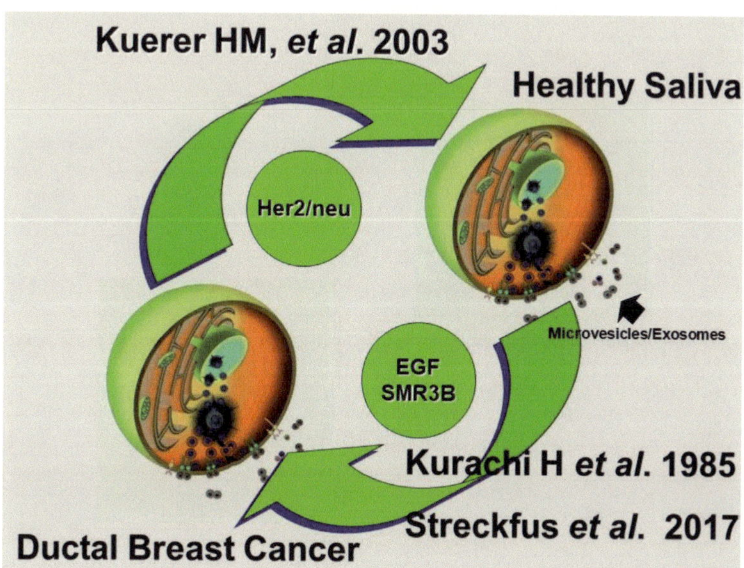

Figure 6.
Feedback systems going from saliva to the tumor [65], from saliva in response to the tumor [48] and from the tumor to healthy breast tissues [66] and saliva [20, 21].

In addition, Kuerer [28] found that healthy contralateral breast aspirates exhibited elevated Her2/neu concentrations secondary to carcinoma in the opposite breast [66]. This supported the findings of Streckfus, where salivary Her2/neu concentrations secondary to carcinoma of the breast [21]. These findings suggest *inter-exocrine gland communication* perhaps by microvesicles and/or exosomes.

Taken together, the author presents sufficient evidence of the interrelationship of exocrine tissues and the possibility of using saliva not only as a diagnostic media, also to study or assess breast cancer progression.

Acknowledgements

This project was supported in part by the R55 DE/OD12414-01 James A. Shannon Director's Award, NIDCR/OD/NIH. The research presented in this manuscript was supported by the Avon Breast Cancer Foundation (#07-2007-071), Komen Foundation (KG080928), Gillson-Longenbaugh Foundation and the Texas Ignition Fund.

The author would like to acknowledge Maija Puhka, Ph.D. of the EV CORE and Institute for Molecular Medicine Finland FIMM University of Helsinki, Finland email: maija.puhka@fimm.fi for the use of the electron micrographic image used in **Figure 3** of this chapter.

Conflict of interest

The author has no conflict of interest or declarations to report.

Thanks

A special note of thanks goes to Lenora G. Bigler, Ph.D. for her more than 20 years of hard work and dedication to this project.

Author details

Charles F. Streckfus
Department of Diagnostic and Biomedical Sciences, University of Texas School of Dentistry at Houston, Houston, TX, United States

*Address all correspondence to: charles.streckfus@uth.tmc.edu

References

[1] Healthy People 2020 [Internet]. Washington, DC: U.S. Department of Health and Human Services, Office of Disease Prevention and Health Promotion, 2019. Available from: https://www.cdc.gov/dhdsp/hp2020.htm

[2] The Breast Cancer Landscape Department of Defense Breast Cancer Research Program. February 2019. Available from: https://cdmrp.army.mil/bcrp/pdfs/Breast%20Cancer%20Landscape.pdf

[3] Bray F, Ferlay J, Soerjomataram I, Siegel RL, Torre LA, Jemal A. Global cancer statistics 2018: GLOBOCAN estimates of incidence and mortality worldwide for 36 cancers in 185 countries. CA: A Cancer Journal for Clinicians. 2018;**68**(6):394-424. DOI: 10.3322/caac.21492

[4] Siegel RL, Miller KD, Jemal A. Cancer statistics, 2019. CA: A Cancer Journal for Clinicians. 2019;**69**(1):7-34. DOI: 10.3322/caac.21551

[5] American Cancer Society. Cancer Facts & Figures 2019. Atlanta: American Cancer Society; 2019

[6] Globocan. Graph Production: Global Cancer Observatory International Agency for Research on Cancer 2018 [cited International Agency for Research on Cancer]. Available from: http://gco.iarc.fr/

[7] SEER*Stat Database: (1975-2012). Bethesda, MD: National Cancer Institute Surveillance Research Program; 2015

[8] Allegra CJ, Aberle DR, Ganschow P, Hahn SM, Lee CN, Millon-Underwood S, et al. NIH state-of-the-science conference statement: Diagnosis and management of ductal carcinoma in situ (DCIS). NIH Consensus and State-of-the-Science Statements. 2009;**26**(2):1-27

[9] Welch HG, Prorok PC, O'Malley AJ, Kramer BS. Breast-cancer tumor size, over-diagnosis, and mammography screening effectiveness. The New England Journal of Medicine. 2016;**375**(15):1347-1438. DOI: 10.1056/NEJMoa1600249

[10] Michaelson JS, Halpern E, Kopans DB. Breast cancer: Computer simulation method for estimating optimal intervals for screening. Radiology. 1999;**212**:551-560

[11] Department of Defense Breast Cancer Research Program. Available from: https://cdmrp.army.mil/pubs/press/2019/19bcrppreann

[12] Thompson A, Brennan K, Cox A, Gee J, Harcourt D, Harris A, et al. Evaluation of the current knowledge limitations in breast cancer research: A gap analysis. Breast Cancer Research. 2008;**10**(2):R26. DOI: 10.1186/bcr1983

[13] Streckfus CF, Romaguera J, Streckfus CE. The use of salivary protein secretions as an in vivo model to study mantel cell lymphoma progression and treatment. Cancer Investigation. 2013;**31**(7):494-499. DOI: 10.3109/07357907.2013.820319

[14] Streckfus CF, Nwizu N, Streckfus CG, Arreola D. Profile of tumor-associated cytokines in breast cancer patients: A preliminary study. Journal of Cancer Science and Clinical Oncology. 2018;**5**(2):206-218

[15] Streckfus CF, Bigler LR. Saliva as a diagnostic fluid. Oral Diseases. 2002;**8**:69-76

[16] Jenzano JW, Courts NF, Timko DA, Lundblad RL. Levels of glandular kallikrein in whole saliva obtained from patients with solid tumors remote from the oral cavity. Journal of Dental Research. 1986;**65**:67-70

[17] Navarro MA, Mesia R, Diez-Gibert O, Rueda A, Ojeda B, Alonso MC. Epidermal growth factor in plasma and saliva of patients with active breast cancer and breast cancer patients in follow-up compared with healthy women. Breast Cancer Research and Treatment. 2009;**42**:83-86

[18] Brooks MN, Wang J, Li Y, Zhang R, Elashoff D, Wong DT. Salivary protein factors are elevated in breast cancer patients. Molecular Medicine Reports. 2008;**1**:375-378

[19] Streckfus C, Bigler L, Dellinger T, Pfeifer M, Rose A, Thigpen J. CA 15-3 and c-erbB-2 presence in the saliva of women. Clinical Oral Investigations. 1999;**3**:138-143

[20] Streckfus C, Bigler L, Tucci M, Thigpen JT. A preliminary study of CA15-3, c-erbB-2, epidermal growth factor receptor, cathepsin-D, and p53 in saliva among women with breast carcinoma. Cancer Investigation. 2000;**18**:101-109

[21] Streckfus C, Bigler L, Dellinger T, Dai X, Kingman A, Thigpen JT. The presence of soluble c-erbB-2 in saliva and serum among women with breast carcinoma: A preliminary study. Clinical Cancer Research. 2000;**6**:2363-2370

[22] Carvajal S, Fera SN, Jones AL, Baldo TA, Mosa IM, Rusling JF, et al. Disposable inkjet-printed electrochemical platform for detection of clinically relevant HER-2 breast cancer biomarker. Biosensors & Bioelectronics. 2018;**1**(104):158-162. DOI: 10.1016/j.bios.2018.01.003

[23] Laidi F, Bouziane A, Errachid A, Zaoui F. Usefulness of salivary and serum auto-antibodies against tumor biomarkers HER2 and MUC1 in breast cancer screening. Asian Pacific Journal of Cancer Prevention. 2016;**17**(1):335-339. DOI: 10.7314/APJCP.2016.17.1.335

[24] Madan Kumar PD, Kandavel S. Salivary human epidermal growth factor receptors 2 levels in patients with different stages of breast cancer: A cross sectional study. Journal of Global Oncology. 2018;**4**(Suppl. 2):55s

[25] Wick MR, Ockner DM, Mills SE, Ritter JH, Swanson PE. Homologous carcinomas of the breasts, skin, and salivary glands. A histologic and immunohistochemical comparison of ductal mammary carcinoma, ductal sweat gland carcinoma and salivary duct carcinoma. American Journal of Clinical Pathology. 1998;**109**:75-84

[26] Nagler RM, Kerner H, Ben-Eliezer S, Minkov I, Ben-Itzhak O. Prognostic role of apoptotic, Bcl-2, c-erbB-2, and p53 tumor markers in salivary gland. Oncology. 2003;**64**:389-398

[27] Breuer B, Smith S, Thor A, Edgerton S, Osborne MP, Minick R, et al. ErbB-2 protein in sera and tumors of breast cancer patients. Breast Cancer Research and Treatment. 1998;**49**:261-270

[28] Kuerer HM, Thompson PA, Krishnamurthy S, Fritsche HA, Marcy SM, Babiera GV, et al. High and differential expression of HER2/neu extracellular domain in bilateral ductal fluids from women with unilateral invasive breast cancer. Clinical Cancer Research. 2003;**9**:601-605

[29] Laidi F, Bouziane A, Lakhdar A, Khabouze S, Rhrab B, Zaoui F. Salivary expression of soluble HER2 in breast cancer patients with positive and negative HER2 status. OncoTargets and Therapy. 2014;**7**:1285-1289. DOI: 10.2147/OTT.564230

[30] McIntyre R, Bigler L, Dellinger T, Pfeifer M, Mannery T, Streckfus C. Oral contraceptive usage and the expression of CA 15-3 and C-erbB-2 in the saliva of healthy women. Oral Surgery, Oral Medicine, Oral Pathology,

Oral Radiology, and Endodontics. 1999;**88**:687-690

[31] Bigler LG, Streckfus CF, Copeland L, Burns R, Dai X, Kuhn M, et al. The potential use of saliva to detect recurrence of disease in women with breast carcinoma. Journal of Oral Pathology & Medicine. 2002;**31**:421-431

[32] Streckfus C, Bigler L, Dellinger T, Dai X, Cox WJ, McArthur A, et al. Reliability assessment of soluble c-erbB-2 concentrations in the saliva of healthy women and men. Oral Surgery, Oral Medicine, Oral Pathology, Oral Radiology, and Endodontics. 2001;**91**:174-179

[33] Streckfus CF, Bigler L, Dellinger T, Kuhn M, Chouinard N, Dai X. The expression of the c-erbB-2 receptor protein in glandular salivary secretions. Journal of Oral Pathology & Medicine. 2004;**33**:595-600

[34] Brinkley J, Copeland L, Streckfus C, Tucci M, Benguzzi H. Sustained delivery of Her-2/neu antibody by TCPL delivery device using adult male rats as a model. Biomedical Sciences Instrumentation. 2003;**39**:324-328

[35] Streckfus C, Bigler LR, Zwick M. The use of surface-enhanced laser desorption/ionization time-of-flight mass spectrometry to detect putative breast cancer markers in saliva: A feasibility study. Journal of Oral Pathology & Medicine. 2006;**35**:292-300

[36] Zabrecky JR, Lam T, Mckenzie SJ, Carney W. The extracellular domain of p185/neu is released from the surface of human breast carcinoma cells, SK-BR-3. The Journal of Biological Chemistry. 1991;**266**:1716-1720

[37] Streckfus CF, Mayorga-Wark O, Daniel Arreola D, Edwards C, Bigler L, Dubinsky WP. Breast cancer related proteins are present in saliva and are modulated secondary to ductal carcinoma in situ of the breast. Cancer Investigation. 2008;**26**(2):159-167

[38] Streckfus CF, Bigler L, Storthz K, Dubinsky WPA. Comparison of the Oncoproteomic profiles in pooled saliva specimens from individuals diagnosed with stage IIa and stage IIb ductal carcinoma of the breast and healthy controls. Journal of Oncology. 2009: 1-12. DOI: 10.1155/2009/7376.19

[39] Streckfus CF, Arreola D, Edwards C, Bigler LA. Comparison of salivary protein profiles between Her2/neu receptor positive and negative breast cancer patients: Support for using salivary protein profiles for modeling breast cancer progression. Journal of Oncology. 2012;**2012**:413256. DOI: 10.1155/2012/413256

[40] Streckfus C, Bigler L. A catalogue of altered salivary proteins secondary to invasive ductal carcinoma: A novel *in vivo* paradigm to assess breast cancer progression. Nature Scientific Reports. 2016;**30800**(6):1-18. DOI: 10.1038/srep30800

[41] Hutchens TW, Yip TT. New desorption strategies for the mass spectrometric analysis of macromolecules. Rapid Communications in Mass Spectrometry. 1993;7:576-580

[42] Merchant M, Weinberger SR. Recent advancements in surface enhanced laser desorption/ionization-time of flight-mass spectrometry. Electrophoresis. 2000;**21**:1164-1177

[43] Madoz-Gurpide J, Wang H, Misek DE, Brichory F, Hanash SM. Protein based microarrays: A tool for probing the proteome of cancer cells and tissues. Proteomics. 2001;**1**:1279-1287

[44] Li J, Zhang Z, Rosenzweig J, Wang YY, Chan D. Proteomics and bioinformatics approaches for identification of serum biomarkers to

detect breast cancer. Clinical Chemistry. 2002;**48**:1296-1304

[45] Arraztio A. Pooling samples for proteomics—Biomarker-profiling case studies. 2014. Available from: http://www.tebu-bio.com/blog/214/07/09/pooling samples for proteomics-biomarker profiling case studies/

[46] Bigler LG, Streckfus CF. A unique protein screening analysis of stimulated whole saliva from normal and breast cancer patients. Preclinica. 2004;**2**(1):52-56

[47] Streckfus CF. Relationship between salivary adiponectin and IGF-1, obesity and breast cancer. Journal of Solid Tumors. 2018;**8**(1):1-9

[48] Streckfus CF, Arreola D, Streckfus CG, Bigler LR. Salivary proline rich peptide decreases cell growth in HCC38 triple negative breast cancer cell line. Journal of Solid Tumors. 2017;**7**(2): 38-44. DOI: 10.5430/jst.v7n2p38

[49] Wood N, Streckfus C. The expression of lung resistance protein in saliva: A novel prognostic indicator protein for carcinoma of the breast. Cancer Investigation. 2015;**33**(10): 510-515. DOI: 10.3109/07357907

[50] Chevalier F, Hirtz C, Chay S, et al. Proteomic studies of saliva: Proposal for a standardized handling of clinical samples. Clinical Proteomics. 2007;**3**: 13-21. DOI: 10.1007/s12014-007-9000-x

[51] Ventura TMDS, Ribeiro NR, Dionizio AS, Sabino IT, Buzalaf MAR. Standardization of a protocol for shotgun proteomic analysis of saliva. Journal of Applied Oral Science. 2018;**26**:e20170561. DOI: 10.1590/1678-7757-2017-0561

[52] Li Y, Zhou X, St John MA, Wong DT. RNA profiling of cell-free saliva using microarray technology. Journal of Dental Research. 2004;**83**(3):199-203

[53] Zhang L, Xiao H, Karan S, Zhou H, Gross J, Elashoff D, et al. Discovery and preclinical validation of salivary transcriptomic and proteomic biomarkers for the detection of breast cancer. PLoS One. 2010;**5**:e15573

[54] Park N, Li Y, Yu T, Brinkman B, Wong D. Characterization of RNA in saliva. Clinical Chemistry. 2006;**52**(6):988-994

[55] Wong DT. Salivary extracellular non-coding RNA: Emerging biomarkers for molecular diagnostics. Journal of Clinical Therapeutics. 2015;**37**(3):540-551. DOI: 10.1016/j.clinthera.2015.02.017

[56] Zhang J, Yang J, Zhang X, Xu J, Sun Y, Zhang P. MicroRNA-10b expression in breast cancer and its clinical association. PLoS One. 2018;**13**(2):e0192509. DOI: 10.1371/journal.pone.0192509

[57] Kirani K, Streckfus CF, Schaefer J. Salivary miRNA as biomarkers to detect breast cancer. IADR Conference; 25 March 2017; San Francisco, CA, ID 4067, JDRa; 2017. Available from: https://iadr.abstractarchives.com/abstract/17iags-2632892/salivary-mirna-in-breast-cancer

[58] Lau CS, Wong DTW. Breast cancer exosome-like microvesicles and salivary gland cells interplay alters salivary gland cell-derived exosome-like microvesicles in vitro. PLoS One. 2012;**7**(3):e33037. DOI: 10.1371/journal.pone.0033037

[59] Han Y, Jia L, Zheng Y, Li W. Salivary exosomes: Emerging roles in systemic disease. International Journal of Biological Sciences. 2018;**14**(6):633-643. DOI: 10.7150/ijbs.25018

[60] Kalra H, Drummen GPC, Mathivanan S. Focus on extracellular vesicles: Introducing the next small big thing. International Journal of Molecular Sciences. 2016;**17**(2):170. DOI: 10.3390/ijms17020170

[61] Lowry MC, Gallagher WM, O'Driscoll L. The role of exosomes in breast cancer. Clinical Chemistry. 2015;**61**(12):1457-1465

[62] Andre F, Schartz N, Movassagh M, Flament C, Pautier P, et al. Malignant effusions and immunogenic tumour-derived exosomes. Lancet (London, England). 2002;**360**(27):295-305

[63] Sugimoto M, Wong DT, Hirayama A, et al. Metabolomics. 2010;**6**:78. DOI: 10.1007/s11306-009-0178-y

[64] Jinno H, Murata T, Sunamura M, Sugimoto H. Investigation of potential salivary biomarkers for the diagnosis of breast cancer. Journal of Clinical Oncology. 2015;**33**(28_suppl):145

[65] Kurachi H, Okamoto S, Oka T. Evidence for the involvement of the submandibular gland epidermal growth factor in mouse mammary tumorigenesis. Proceedings of the National Academy of Sciences of the United States of America. 1985;**82**:5940-5943

[66] Kuerer HM, Thompson PA, Krishnamurthy S, Fritsche HA, Marcy SM, et al. High and differential expression of HER-2/neu extracellular domain in bilateral ductal fluids from women with unilateral invasive breast cancer. Clinical Cancer Research. 2003;**9**(2):601-605

Chapter 6

Advantages of Salivary DNA in Human Identification

Raluca Dumache, Veronica Ciocan, Camelia Muresan, Ramona Parvanescu and Alexandra Enache

Abstract

Since two and a half decades, in human identification, the short tandem repeat (STR) markers represent the "gold standard." Besides them, haploid markers such as X-STR and Y-STR are also used to complement the autosomal markers. In human identification, DNA from body fluids, especially saliva, represents an important tool. The aim of this chapter is to present the importance of analyzing X-STR markers in a relatedness case between a sister and her presumptive brother, a carbonized victim using body fluids for their DNA identification. Our laboratory had to establish the relatedness between a woman and her presumptive brother (PB), who was the victim of a car accident explosion. In this case, as reference sample we used saliva collected on swabs from the woman and blood sample from the deceased victim. For the DNA extraction, DNA IQ Casework (Promega, USA) was used. DNA quantification was done with PowerQuant System kit (Promega, USA). Furthermore, the DNA samples were amplified with Investigator 24plex QS (Qiagen, Germany) for the STR markers and Investigator Argus 12-X QS kit (Qiagen, Germany) for the X-STR markers. The amplified DNA products were separated by capillary electrophoresis on a 3500 Genetic Analyzer. In this case, full genetic profiles were obtained for the woman and her presumptive brother on both STR and X-STR markers. Thus, we could confirm a full sibling relationship between them. Since the introduction of DNA in human identification, it represents a useful tool in establishing sibling relationship from different biological samples.

Keywords: saliva, deoxyribonucleic acid (DNA), short tandem repeat (STR) markers, X-STR markers, PCR (polymerase chain reaction), capillary electrophoresis (CE)

1. Introduction

A few years ago, the FBI Laboratory announced the expansion of the common core of 13 STR markers included in the National DNA Index System (NDIS) since 1997. Starting with 1st of January 2017, FBI required the CODIS (Combined DNA Index System) laboratories to implement additional STR markers [1]. The new markers added to the common core of 13 STR markers aid in human identification and in kinship analysis of missing persons due to a better power of discrimination [2]. In order to confirm the identity of a person, it is necessary to perform a comparative study of DNA profiles belonging to that person and a first-degree relative (mother/father; brother-sister), in which the respecting of the classical laws for transmitting the hereditary characters is followed, so that a maternal allele and a paternal allele are found on a DNA locus [3, 4]. Within a paternity investigation, the child's mother being presumed as being certain, the child's DNA profile presents a lot of alleles that are found in the presumptive father profile besides the maternal alleles; we can speak about a confirmation of paternity that is always expressed in probability terms. In cases where the biological parents do not exist anymore, a sibling or cousin is recommended to participate in the DNA identification process [5–7]. In DNA human identification, body fluids such as saliva, blood, semen, and urine represent important components. Regarding saliva, it can be obtained easily, by non-invasive techniques through the buccal swabbing. Herein, we present the importance of salivary DNA and STR markers and haploid markers in establishing the identity of a carbonized corpse through DNA sibling analysis.

2. Materials and methods

2.1 DNA extraction from the biological samples

For the reference samples of the victim's sister, we collected epithelial cells from the inner cheeks on three buccal swabs (Copan, Italy) [8]. In case of the carbonized victim, during the autopsy procedure, we collected blood samples from the heart chambers in collection tubes with EDTA. In this case of kinship analysis, the saliva was collected by swabbing from the inner cheeks of the woman. In cases of carbonized corpses, depending on their grade of carbonization, the biological samples used for the identification by DNA analysis can be saliva obtained from the mouth and blood obtained from the heart chambers or different parts of the internal organs.

The swabs from the victim's sister were left to dry for 3–4 h in a laminar PCR flow hood. Following the recommendations of the manufacturer, we proceeded to the DNA extraction from the saliva and blood. The DNA extraction was performed by the automated Maxwell® 16 RSC instrument (Promega, USA) using the Maxwell® RSC Whole Blood DNA kit (Promega, USA) for the blood samples and the Maxwell RSC Buccal Swab DNA kit (Promega, USA) for the swabs [9].

2.2 Quantification of the extracted DNA samples

For the quantification of the DNA samples from the woman and her presumptive brother, PowerQuant System kit (Promega, USA) [10] was used. In this case, following the manufacturer's recommendations, we prepared a mix solution for each sample with a final volume of 18 μL consisting of 10 μL of PowerQuant 2× Master Mix; 7 μL of amplification grade (water), and 1 μL of Power Quant 20× Primer Mix. The quantification was made on a 7500 real time PCR (Applied Biosystems, USA), using the HID Real-Time PCR Analysis Software v 2.0.6. The concentrations of saliva and blood are presented in **Table 1**.

Person's identity	Concentrations (ng/μL)
Sister	1.08
Presumptive brother	3.25

Table 1.
DNA concentrations of the woman and her presumptive brother.

3. Amplification of the DNA samples

The DNA samples from the woman and her alleged brother were amplified for the STR markers using the Investigator 24plex QS kit (Qiagen, Germany) [11]. Also, in this case, the X-STR markers have been analyzed using the Investigator Argus 12-X-QS kit (Qiagen, Germany) [12]. All these genetic markers are contained in a single reaction, known as multiplex. For the STR markers, a number of 23 STR markers were investigated, and for the X-STR markers, a number of 12 markers were analyzed. The analysis was done after the recommendations of the manufacturers.

3.1 Amplification of the autosomal STR markers

In this step, the DNA sample's amplification was performed on a ProFlex PCR System (Applied Biosystems, USA). We used the Investigator 24plex QS Kit (Qiagen, Germany). Furthermore, the PCR reactions of the salivary DNA samples were carried out in a total volume of 25 μL. The final volume of the reaction contained Fast Reaction Mix 2.0: 7.5 μL, Primer Mix: 2.5 μL, nuclease-free water: 12.5 μL, and template DNA: 2.5 μL.

The Investigator 24plex QS Kit (Qiagen, Germany) contains 23 autosomal markers, as follows: D1S1656, D2S441, D2S1338, D3S1358, D5S818, D7S820, D8S1179, D10S1248, D12S391, D13S317, D16S539, D18S51, D19S433, D21S11, D22S1045, CSF1PO, FGA, TH01, TPOX, Vwa, SE33, DYS391, and amelogenin. All these genetic markers are contained in a single reaction, known as multiplex. The conditions for the PCR amplification were as follows:

- 3 PCR cycles: temperature (T) = 98°C for 30 s; T = 64°C for 55 s; T = 72°C for 5 s;

- 27 PCR cycles: T = 96°C for 10 s; T = 61°C for 55 s; T = 72°C for 5 s.

After 30 PCR cycles were completed, a final extension (hold) at T = 68°C for 2 min followed by final hold indefinite at T = 10°C.

3.2 Amplification of the X-STR markers

In this case, because we have a brother-sister relationship, we amplified the X-STR markers using the Investigator Argus 12-X QS kit (Qiagen, Germany). The kit contains 12 X-STR markers as follows: DXS8378, DXS10135, DXS10148, DXS7132, DXS10074, DXS10079, XPRTB, DXS10101, DXS10103, DXS7423, DXS10134, and DXS10146.

The final reaction volume contained: Fast Reaction Mix 2.0: 7.5 μL; Primer Mix: 2.5 μL; nuclease-free water: 12.5 μL, and template DNA: 2.5 μL.

The amplification conditions for X-STRs were as follows in the cycling protocol:

- 3 PCR cycles as follows: T = 98°C for 60 s; T = 61°C for 100 s; T = 72°C for 5 s.

- 27 PCR cycles as follows: T = 96°C for 10 s; T = 61°C for 100 s and T = 72°C for 5 s.

After 30 PCR cycles were completed, a final extension (hold) at T = 68°C for 2 min followed by final hold indefinite at T = 10°C.

4. Capillary electrophoresis of the amplified DNA samples

For the capillary electrophoresis, the samples were analyzed on a 3500 Genetic Analyzer, following the manufacturer's recommendations. For the STR markers, we used 1 μL of the amplified PCR product (DNA sample) and the allelic ladder (AL). They were added into the mix containing: 12.5 μL of Hi-Di formamide (Applied Biosystems, USA) and 0.5 μL DNA size standard BTO (Qiagen, Germany). To analyze the X-STR markers, we added 1 μL of the amplified PCR product (DNA sample) and the allelic ladder (AL) into the mix containing: 12.5 μL of Hi-Di formamide (Qiagen, Germany) and 0.5 μL DNA size standard BTO (Qiagen, Germany). Gene Mapper ID-X Software version 1.4 (Applied Biosystems, USA) was used to analyze the obtained data [13].

5. Results

After the DNA separation, we obtained the electropherograms and the genotypes of the unidentified person and his alleged brothers using the Gene Mapper ID-X software version 1.4 (Applied Biosystems, USA). GenoProof 3 Software-Kinship Examination (Qualitype GmbH, Dresden, Germany) [14] was used for the statistical part. In this case, a full sibling probability of 99.999972% was obtained between the woman and her presumptive brother. Also, because they had a sibling relationship as brother-sister, we analyzed the X-STR markers. The genetic profiles on STR markers between the woman and her presumptive brother are presented in **Figures 1** and **2**, respectively. X-STR haplotypes on the woman and her presumptive brother are presented in **Figures 3** and **4**, respectively.

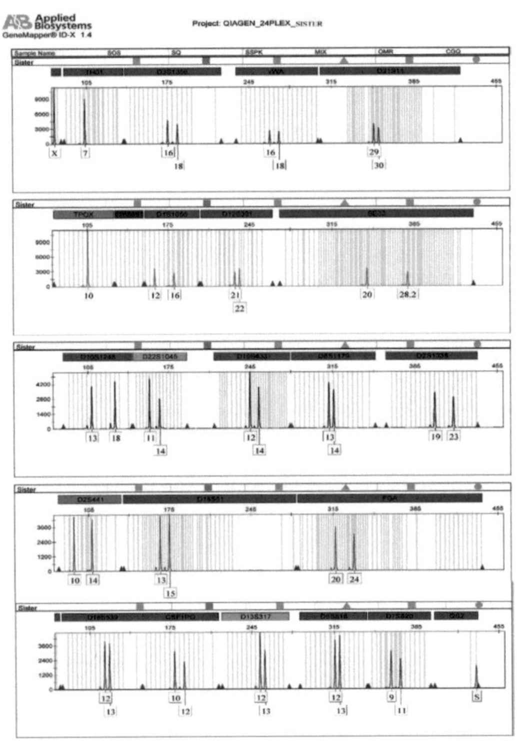

Figure 1.
Woman's genetic profile on 23 STR markers.

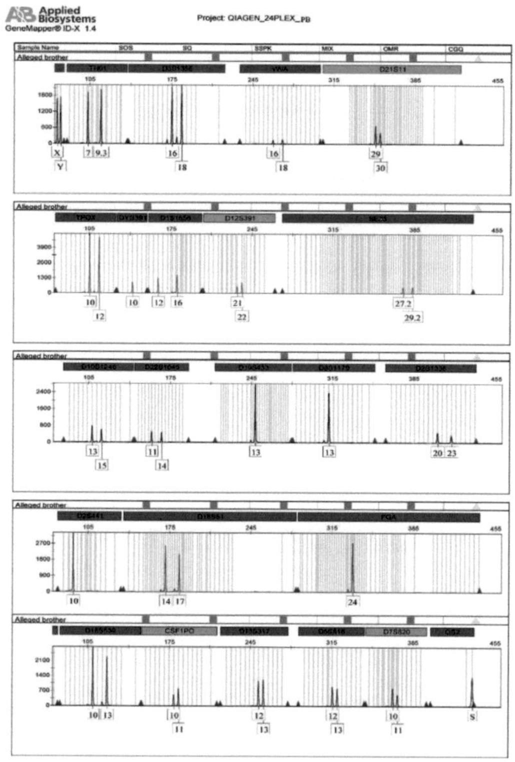

Figure 2.
Genetic profile of the presumptive brother on 23 STR markers.

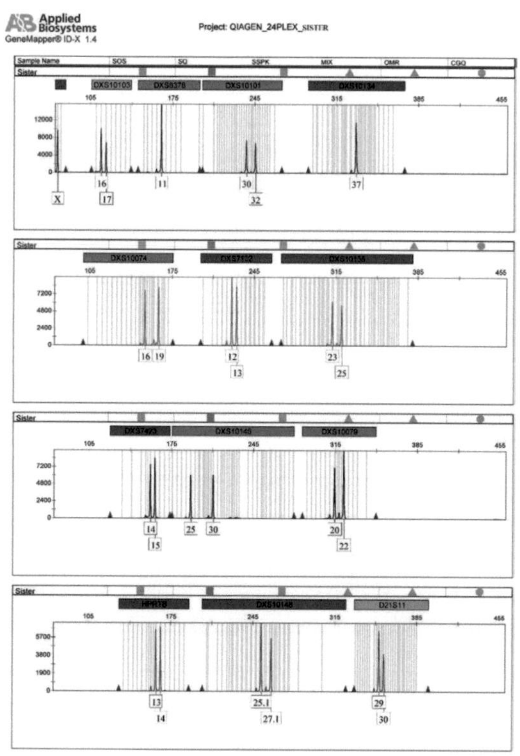

Figure 3.
X-STR haplotype of the woman.

The genetic profiles of the woman and her presumptive brother on X-STR markers are presented in **Table 2**.

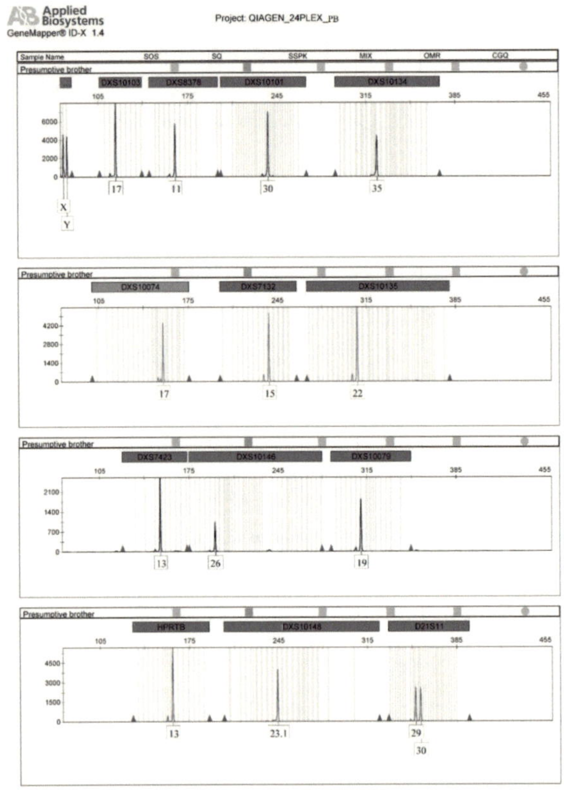

Figure 4.
X-STR haplotype of the presumptive brother.

X MARKER	Sister	Common genes	Presumptive Brother
DXS8378	11	-	10
DXS10135	20;30	-	23.1
DXS10148	25.1	25.1	25.1
DXS7132	14	14	14
DXS10074	18;19		16
DXS10079	19	19	19
HPRTB	13;14	-	12
DXS10101	28.2;32	-	24;29.2
DXS10103	16;19	-	20
DXS7423	14;15	-	16
DXS10134	36;37	36	36
DXS10146	28	-	29
D21S11	30;33.2	-	30;33.2

Note: The 4 colors represent the dyes. The markers are divided into 4 linkage groups (3 markers per group).

Table 2.
Common X-STR markers between the woman and her presumptive brother.

6. Discussions

Saliva as a body fluid is very often used in laboratory tests for diagnosis, prevention, and monitoring of different diseases. Compered to blood tests, saliva tests present some advantages like easy and non-invasive collection techniques; its collection does not present any risks for the technician who collects the samples.

In the future, salivary DNA diagnostic tests can eliminate the blood tests, because the DNA contains the same genetic information from all the biological samples.

Also, in forensic human identification, salivary DNA has improved the laboratory workflow because it is easily collected and can be quickly analyzed by direct PCR method. After collecting saliva on buccal swab or FTA paper, the sample can be directly amplified by polymerase chain reaction (PCR) in less than an hour, followed by migration on capillary electrophoresis.

7. Conclusions

In human identification from DNA, establishing the paternity or maternity, sibling or kinship analysis can be done from body fluids, by non-invasive collection techniques. In this chapter, we presented the usefulness of both saliva and blood in a case of sibling relationship.

Conflict of interest

The authors declare they have no conflict of interest.

Author details

Raluca Dumache[1,3]*, Veronica Ciocan[1,2], Camelia Muresan[1,2], Ramona Parvanescu[3,4] and Alexandra Enache[1,2]

1 Faculty of Medicine, Victor Babes University of Medicine and Pharmacy, Timisoara, Romania

2 Institute of Forensic Medicine, Timisoara, Romania

3 Laboratory of Forensic Genetics, Victor Babes University of Medicine and Pharmacy, Timisoara, Romania

4 Doctoral School of Victor Babes University of Medicine and Pharmacy, Timisoara, Romania

*Address all correspondence to: raluca.dumache@umft.ro

References

[1] Hares DR. Selection and implementation of expanded CODIS core loci in the United States. Forensic Science International: Genetics. 2015;**17**:33-34

[2] Davis C, Ge J, King J, Malik N, et al. Variants observed for STR locus SE33: A concordance study. Forensic Science International: Genetics. 2012;**6**:494-497

[3] Diegoli TM. Forensic typing of short tandem repeat markers on the X and Y chromosomes. Forensic Science International: Genetics. 2015;**18**:140-151

[4] Pereira V, Tomas C, Amorim A, Morling N, Gusmao L, Prata MJ. Study of 25 X-chromosome SNPs in the Portuguese. Forensic Science International: Genetics. 2011;**5**:336-338

[5] Szibor R, Krawczak M, Hering S, Edelmann J, Kuhlisch E, et al. Use of X-linked markers for forensic purposes. International Journal of Legal Medicine. 2003;**117**:67-74

[6] Toscanini U, Berardi G, Gomez A, Raimondi E. X-STRs analysis in paternity testing when the alleged father is related to the biological father. Forensic Science International: Genetics Supplement Series. 2009;**2**:234-235

[7] Illescas MJ, Aznar JM, Cardoso S, Lopez-Oceja A, Gammara D, Sanchez-Romerra JF, et al. Genetic characterization of ten X-STRs in a population from Spanish Levant. Forensic Science International: Genetics. 2012;**6**:e180-e181

[8] Available from: https://www.promega.ro/products/genetic-identity/genetic-identity-workflow/dna-isolation/dna-iq-system/?catNum=DC6701

[9] Available from: https://www.promega.ro/resources/protocols/technical-manuals/101/maxwell-rsc-instrument-operating-manual-protocol/

[10] Bright JA, Curran JM, Buckleton JS. Relatedness calculations for linked loci incorporating subpopulation effects. Forensic Science International: Genetics. 2013;**7**:380-383

[11] Szibor R. X-chromosomal markers: Past, present, future. Forensic Science International: Genetics. 2007;**1**:93-99

[12] Turrina S, Atzei R, Filipinni G, De Leo D. Development and forensic validation of the new multiplex PCR assay with 12 X-chromosomal short tandem repeats. Forensic Science International: Genetics. 2007;**1**:201-224

[13] Elakkary S, Hoffmeister-Ullerich S, Schultze C, Seif E, Sheta A, Hering S, et al. Genetic polymorphisms of the twelve X-STRs of the investigator Argus X-12 kit and additional six X-STR centromere region loci in an Egyptian population sample. Forensic Science International: Genetics. 2014;**11**:26-30

[14] Dumache R, Rogobete AF, Ciocan V, Muresan C, Enache A. DNA-based identification of a carbonized victim by kinship analysis. Clinical Laboratory. 2017;**63**:1035-1040